04/2019

BOWEN ISLAND LIBRARY

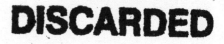
3 0947 0005 5442 4

DISCARDED

# MINDFULNESS FOR ALL

D0391768

Bowen Island Public Library

DISCARDED

ALSO BY JON KABAT-ZINN

*MEDITATION IS NOT WHAT YOU THINK: Mindfulness and
Why It Is So Important*
*FALLING AWAKE: How to Practice Mindfulness in Everyday Life*
*THE HEALING POWER OF MINDFULNESS: A New Way of Being*

*MINDFULNESS:*
*Diverse Perspectives on Its Meaning, Origins, and Applications*
(editor, with J. Mark G. Williams)

*MINDFULNESS FOR BEGINNERS:*
*Reclaiming the Present Moment—and Your Life*

*THE MIND'S OWN PHYSICIAN:*
*A Scientific Dialogue with the Dalai Lama on the Healing Power of Meditation*
(editor, with Richard J. Davidson)

*LETTING EVERYTHING BECOME YOUR TEACHER:*
*100 Lessons in Mindfulness*

*ARRIVING AT YOUR OWN DOOR:*
*108 Lessons in Mindfulness*

*THE MINDFUL WAY THROUGH DEPRESSION:*
*Freeing Yourself from Chronic Unhappiness*
(with Mark Williams, John Teasdale, and Zindel Segal)

*COMING TO OUR SENSES:*
*Healing Ourselves and the World Through Mindfulness*

*EVERYDAY BLESSINGS:*
*The Inner Work of Mindful Parenting*
(with Myla Kabat-Zinn)

*WHEREVER YOU GO, THERE YOU ARE:*
*Mindfulness Meditation in Everyday Life*

*FULL CATASTROPHE LIVING:*
*Using the Wisdom of Your Body and Mind to Face Stress, Pain, and Illness*

Bowen Island Public Library

# MINDFULNESS FOR ALL

## *The Wisdom to Transform the World*

JON KABAT-ZINN

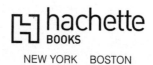
hachette
**BOOKS**

NEW YORK  BOSTON

Copyright © 2019 by Jon Kabat-Zinn, Ph.D.

Cover design by Joanne O'Neill
Cover copyright © 2019 by Hachette Book Group, Inc.

Hachette Book Group supports the right to free expression and the value of copyright. The purpose of copyright is to encourage writers and artists to produce the creative works that enrich our culture.

The scanning, uploading, and distribution of this book without permission is a theft of the author's intellectual property. If you would like permission to use material from the book (other than for review purposes), please contact permissions@hbgusa.com. Thank you for your support of the author's rights.

Hachette Books
Hachette Book Group
1290 Avenue of the Americas
New York, NY 10104
hachettebooks.com
twitter.com/hachettebooks

Originally published in hardcover as part of *Coming to Our Senses* by Hyperion in January 2005.

First Edition: February 2019

Credits and permissions appear beginning on p. 149 and constitute a continuation of the copyright page.

Hachette Books is a division of Hachette Book Group, Inc.
The Hachette Books name and logo are trademarks of Hachette Book Group, Inc.

The publisher is not responsible for websites (or their content) that are not owned by the publisher.

The Hachette Speakers Bureau provides a wide range of authors for speaking events. To find out more, go to www.hachettespeakersbureau.com or call (866) 376-6591.

Library of Congress Control Number: 2018957304

ISBNs: 978-0-316-41177-6 (trade paperback), 978-0-316-52203-8 (ebook)

Printed in the United States of America

LSC-C

10 9 8 7 6 5 4 3 2 1

for Myla
for Tayo, Stella, Asa, and Toby
for Will and Teresa
for Naushon
for Serena
for the memory of Sally and Elvin
and Howie and Roz


for all those who care

for what is possible

for what is so

for wisdom

for clarity

for kindness

for love

# CONTENTS

# FOREWORD

Mindfulness for all!

That is a wild thought.

But why not, when you come right down to it? Especially at this moment in time, stressed as we are individually and collectively in so many different ways, both inwardly and outwardly.

And in terms of the wisdom to transform the world, it is not hyperbole. That wisdom is a potential that is wholly distributive, lying within each one of us in small but, as I hope to make clear, hardly insignificant ways. That wisdom is cultivatable through mindfulness in ways both little and big. I have had the privilege of seeing it emerge and flourish in many different domains over the past forty years. Now, that incipient wisdom is spreading throughout the world, becoming stronger and ever more an imperative.

## The Evolutionary Import of Meditative Awareness

If it is part of the evolutionary glide path of us humans to progressively know ourselves better, thereby inhabiting a bit more the name we gave our species\*; if it is also part of the evolutionary glide path of us humans not to destroy ourselves or create nightmare dystopias beyond those we have already managed to perpetrate, we will need to take on a whole new level of responsibility for ourselves, for our own

---

\* *Homo sapiens sapiens*: The species that is aware and knows that it is aware, from the Latin, *sapere,* to taste or to know (see Book 1 in this series, page 131).

minds, for our societies, and for our planet. Otherwise, if past is any prologue, all of us may unwittingly be contributing either by omission or commission, in tiny ways that may not be so tiny in the end, to creating a highly unhealthy and majorly toxic world that none of us will be happy to inhabit. And that is perhaps the understatement of the millennium. The prevailing dis-ease of humanity is playing itself out increasingly before our very eyes. It is also increasingly harder for any of us to ignore, and we do so individually and collectively at our peril.

So mindfulness for all and the cultivation of greater enacted wisdom in how we conduct ourselves and take care of our world is hardly mere hype or wishful thinking. It may be *an*, if not *the*, essential ingredient for our short- and long-term survival, health, and ongoing development as a species. But to be up to the enormity of this challenge, the mindfulness I am referring to has to be authentic, nested within a universal dharma framework nurturing and cultivating wisdom and compassion.* As I am using the term, mindfulness is a way of seeing and a way of being, one that has a long history on this planet. It also has considerable momentum at the moment as it moves increasingly into the mainstream of many different societies and cultures in a variety of ways. Axiomatically, the approach I am advocating has to be and *is* grounded and safeguarded at every level in ethical, embodied, enacted, and ultimately selfless wisdom and action. We might think of mindfulness as one tributary of the human wisdom tradition. While its most articulated roots lie deep within Buddhism, its essence is universal and has been expressed in one way or another in all human cultures and traditions.

As I see it, the increasingly widespread adoption and practice of mindfulness meditation in our individual lives and in our work, and its intentional application moment by moment and day by day in how we respond to the world we inhabit, could potentially provide the very root of authentic well-being, peacefulness, and clarity within

---

* See Book 1: *Meditation Is Not What You Think: Mindfulness and Why It Is So Important* if the word *dharma* is unfamiliar to you.

our vast diversity of peoples, cultures, and aspirations on the planet. Mindfulness has something to offer all of us as individuals, and as a global human community. I don't think that there is any question that its transformative potential needs to be realized—i.e., made real— in an infinite number of creative ways at this particular juncture in the unfolding of our species, nested within our far-more-fragile-than-we-thought-until-recently planetary abode.

As one of many recent indications that mindfulness is moving into the mainstream in broadly influential ways, the very last chapter of the historian Yuval Noah Harari's *21 Lessons for the 21st Century* is about mindfulness. In it, he discloses that since a ten-day retreat in the year 2000, he has been meditating every day, plus annually participating in an intensive silent meditation retreat of one or two months duration (with no books or social media during that time).* That alone tells us a lot. After offering us two remarkably popular, profound, provocative, and insightful volumes describing the history of the human condition† and the challenges we are facing as a species in the very near future,‡ some of them quite terrifying, his most recent work, also a bestseller, distills from all that scholarly investigation twenty-one key lessons for the present. I found it quite revealing and gratifying that, with all the threads Harari so skillfully weaves together from history to reveal the enormous challenges our species is facing now, he explicitly adopts the rigorous practice of mindfulness in his own life and names it as an improbable but perhaps essential element for cultivation if, as a species, we are to thread the needle going forward in facing the new challenges brought on by both information technology and biotechnology, challenges he elaborates in considerable and sobering detail.

When *21 Lessons for the 21st Century* was reviewed on the front page of the Sunday *New York Times Book Review* on September 9,

---

* https://en.wikipedia.org/wiki/Yuval_Noah_Harari
† *Sapiens: A Brief History of Humankind,* HarperCollins, New York, 2015.
‡ *Homo Deus: A Brief History of Tomorrow,* HarperCollins, New York, 2017.

2018, by Bill Gates, under the title, "Thinking Big,"* because Harari is nothing if not a deep and creative thinker and synthesizer as an historian, Gates asks:

> What does Harari think we should do about all this? [i.e., the large challenges Harari enumerates we are facing as a species at this moment in time] Sprinkled throughout is some practical advice, including a three-prong strategy for fighting terrorism and a few tips for dealing with fake news. But his big idea boils down to this: Meditate. Of course he isn't suggesting that the world's problems will vanish if enough of us start sitting in the lotus position and chanting *om*. But he does insist that life in the 21st Century demands mindfulness—getting to know ourselves better and seeing how we contribute to suffering in our own lives. This is easy to mock, but as someone who's taken a course on mindfulness and meditation, I found it compelling.

This is a rather remarkable statement, especially coming from Bill Gates. Apparently he understands the power of mindfulness from the inside.

*

The way I would put the basic message of this book is that before we give up being human in the face of what is very likely on the horizon, i.e. artificial intelligence, intelligent robots, and the prospect of digitally if not also biologically "enhanced" humans, and much more, as Harari

---

* Ironic, in that mindfulness is so much bigger than thinking and orthogonal to it. Awareness and thought are obviously not mutually exclusive at all, and if understood correctly, can complement and benefit each other enormously. In this context, "orthogonal" means that mindfulness, or awareness, is an independent domain or dimension, pertaining at the same time as thinking and able to provide a different vantage point from which to hold all thought. See Book 3, pp. 38–51 for more on orthogonality.

describes in great detail, we might do well to explore in depth what being fully human, and thus, more embodied and more awake might really mean and feel like. That is both the plea and the challenge of this book, and of all four books in the *Coming to Our Senses* series. But it is inviting a very personal engagement on your part, in the sense that each one of us has a responsibility, not only to ourself but to the world, to do our own inner and outer work through the regular cultivation of mindfulness—as a meditation practice and as a way of being—and thereby come to recognize and inhabit the full dimensionality of our being and its repertoire of potentials right here and right now, as best we can.

Since elements of the universal mindfulness meditation-based dharma perspective I am referring to run through wisdom streams within every human culture, mindfulness is intrinsically inclusive, capable of dissolving barriers to communication and finding common purpose rather than promoting divisiveness. There is no one right way to cultivate it and no catechism or belief system one has to adopt. What is more, this emerging wisdom perspective is continuing to evolve through us and through how we choose to lead our lives and face our very real challenges and opportunities. It reflects what has always been deepest and best in us as human beings, in our diversity and in our commonality.

## Befriending Your Own Mind and Body: A Universal Meditation Practice

Of course, the kind of wisdom we are speaking of has to be grounded in ongoing *cultivation*, and that means in a practice of some kind that nurtures, sustains, and deepens it. For mindfulness is not mindfulness if it is not *lived*. And that means *embodied*. Those of us who undertake it in this way do so as best we can—not as an ideal, but as an ongoing and continually unfolding way of being.

Why?

Because mindfulness is not merely a good idea, or a nice philosophy, belief system, or catechism. It is a rigorous universally applicable meditation practice—universal because awareness itself could be seen as the final common pathway of our humanity, across all cultures. When all is said and done, mindfulness is really a way of being— a way of being in relationship to experience. By its very nature, it requires ongoing cultivation and nurturance by us as individuals if we care about living our lives fully and freely, and ultimately, as supportive and nurturing communities and societies. In the same way that musicians need to tune, retune, and fine-tune their instruments on a regular basis before and sometimes even during performances, mindfulness practice can be thought of as a kind of tuning of the instrument of your attention and how you choose to be in relationship to experience—any experience, all experience. It doesn't matter how accomplished a musician you are. You still have to tune your instrument regularly. And the more accomplished you are, the more you need to practice. It is a virtuous circle.

Even the greatest musicians practice. In fact, they probably practice more than anyone else. Only with mindfulness, there is no separation between "rehearsal" and "performance." Why? Because there is no performance, and no rehearsal either. There is only this moment. This is it. There is no "improving" on our awareness. What we are cultivating through the practice of mindfulness is greater *access* to and intimacy with our innate capacity for awareness, and an ability to take up residency, so to speak, in that domain of being as our "default mode," out of which flows all our doing.

## Many Doors, One Room:
### Diversity and Inclusiveness are Paramount

The practice and larger expression of mindfulness in the world needs to be as diverse as the constituencies that might advocate for it, adopt it, embody it, and benefit from it—each in their own way, just as the music played and enjoyed by the human family is so profoundly diverse, a veritable universe of lived expression and connection.

At the same time, if you ask if I am concerned with the hype associated with mindfulness in the world these days, and with the tendency of some to advertise themselves as "mindfulness teachers" without much, if any, grounding in rigorous practice and study, you bet I am. Might the title of this book be contributing to that hype? I certainly hope not. I have been engaged for decades in the endeavor to bring mindfulness into the mainstream of the world in ways that are true to its dharma roots and do not denature or diminish it, precisely because of my conviction about and personal experience (limited as that might be, being just one person) of its profound healing and transformative potential, its widespread applicability, and its many-times-over documented contribution to health and wellbeing at every level that those words carry meaning. And the scientific study of mindfulness, while still in its infancy—although far less so than twenty years ago—is substantiating that there are many different applications of mindfulness beyond MBSR (mindfulness-based stress reduction) and MBCT (mindfulness-based cognitive therapy) in medicine and clinical psychology that are making significant contributions in various domains, including all levels of education, criminal justice, business, sports, community-building, even politics.

Do I mean by "mindfulness for all" that everybody is all of a sudden going to adopt or ultimately wind up with a rigorous and personally meaningful meditation practice? No. Of course not. Still, and highly improbably from the perspective of 1979, when MBSR was first developed in the Stress Reduction Clinic at the University of Massachusetts Medical Center, more and more people around the world and increasingly among diverse and divergent communities *are* actually incorporating consistent and regular mindfulness meditation practice to one degree or another into their lives, from refugees in South Sudan to U.S. Forest Service firefighters, from children in well-researched public school and afterschool programs in inner city Baltimore to cops in major police departments, from people attending drop-in weekly public meditations throughout the city of Los Angeles offered by UCLA's

Mindful Awareness Research Center to medical patients participating in mindfulness programs sponsored by the mindfulness initiative within the Shanghai Medical Society, from the work of affiliate programs of the Center for Mindfulness in Medicine, Health Care, and Society around the world to a far broader world-wide network of MBSR teachers and teacher-trainers in university and hospital centers and stand-alone programs. Mindfulness is taking root on all continents with the possible exception of Antarctica: in North America, Europe, Africa, Asia, and Latin America.

But if you ask whether I mean by that phrase, mindfulness for all, that we could all, as unique human beings, young and old, whoever we are, whatever we do, whatever views we hold, however we have been shaped by the past and our various heritage streams, whatever groups we identify with or belong to—religious, spiritual, or philosophical, secular or sacred, right or left, pessimistic or optimistic, cynical or large of heart—benefit from greater awareness of, in Bill Gate's words, "how we contribute to suffering in our own lives" and, of course, in the lives of others as well; and how we can all benefit from greater wakefulness, greater awareness of our interconnectedness with each other, of the web of life on this planet and within the universe we inhabit, and from recognizing and realizing the essential impersonal non-self nature of all phenomena,* including us, the answer is an emphatic "yes." You bet I do. In fact, I think it could be the most important evolutionary opportunity for humanity at this moment in time, namely to know ourselves in our wholeness and our interconnectedness as a species, and to be able to act out of the wisdom of a larger wholeness rather than out of a more small-minded and often fear-based and misconstrued sense of self-interest and limited and limiting narratives about who we truly are as living breathing beings, here for such a short period on this planet—a full human lifespan, if we are lucky, the blink of an eye in cosmological, or geological, or evolutionary time.

---

* See Book 1, "Emptiness"

## If You Are Human and You Suffer, This Practice May Be for You

And just to bring it to the personal level for a moment, why would you have even had the impulse to pick up this book if you were not in some way intuitively drawn to that very possibility in yourself and for yourself at some level? I am guessing that this is the case even if you weren't and aren't quite sure that you yourself could possibly begin or maintain and nurture your own personal meditation practice over days, weeks, months, years, and decades. The fact is, though, that you can. You can develop your own personal meditation practice in a way that works for you. And more and more of us on this planet are. All you need to do is begin, to put your toe in the water, which you already have if you have read even this far. If what I am saying here is true, the rest will take care of itself . . . life will wind up teaching you, nurturing you in ways you may have not realized were possible, but will come to recognize and appreciate as you do wake up a bit more through the cultivation of moment-to-moment nonjudgmental awareness.

## Life Is the Ultimate Meditation Teacher

The practice of mindfulness ultimately comes down to how you choose to live your life moment by moment by moment while you still have the chance. And more specifically, it is in how you choose to live it in relationship to whatever you may be encountering in terms of what I sometimes call the full catastrophe of the human condition and, closer to home, the sometime full catastrophe of our own individual lives.

In terms of the hype, perhaps it might be valuable for us to back away from the word "mindfulness" for a moment. Mindfulness is just a word. We are pointing to something underneath the word itself, to its deepest significance, namely pure awareness—perhaps humanity's most remarkable feature and evolutionary asset.

Once we are in the domain of pure awareness, we are also in the domain of *relationality*. Precisely because you are paying attention, it becomes a lot easier to see how everything is related to everything else in this interconnected universe. Our challenge, being intrinsically capable of inhabiting our own awareness as our default mode, as well as capable of being *aware* of our own awareness, is this: How are we going to interface with reality itself inwardly and outwardly, in both the domain of being (wakefulness) and the domain of doing (taking action)? Once you tap into and learn to inhabit your own awareness, there is no going back to sleep. And who would want to?

Mindfulness is and always has been also a matter of "heartful-ness." The word for "mind" and the word for heart in Chinese and in many other Asian languages is the same word. In Chinese, the ideogram for mindfulness consists of the character for "presence" or "now" above the character for "heart." So "mindfulness" is "heartful-ness." It always has been. And that means that it is intrinsically ethi-cal. It is and has to be grounded in non-harming. Why? Because it is not possible to be equanimous, at peace in your own heart, if you are engaged in harming or killing others, or lying, or stealing, or in sexual misconduct, or speaking ill of others. All of these are the opposite of non-harming, and of basic human kindness.

## A Rose by Any Other Name...

By the same token, we could also say that mindfulness is, to coin a phrase, in a profound way also "kindfulness." If we called mindful-ness "kindfulness," would anybody object? Would kindfulness seem difficult or beyond our reach, or overly hyped? I doubt it. An act of authentic kindness is usually spontaneous and generous. It comes out of a momentary perceiving of a need and responding in a friendly fashion out of an impulse to connect and perhaps to help. But preced-ing that impulse is a moment of nonconceptual *recognition*, a spon-taneous recognition, before thinking arises, that something is being called out of us, if perhaps simply a smile directed at another in a critical moment, or something more, perhaps an unseen act of generosity directed at another. That recognition is an unbidden moment of discernment, coming out of awareness itself. That *is* mindfulness.

The initiating event could be anything that engenders a heartfelt and heartful response in that moment, whether it involves a loved one, perhaps a child of yours, or for that matter, a homeless person on the street or the person in the car next to you in traffic. It is not the act itself that is most important. It is the *recognition*. And that capacity for recognition is innate. It is intrinsically human. That moment of recognition is a moment of spontaneous mindfulness. It is a moment of nonseparation. It is not mediated by thought, although it can be amplified and rounded out by thought later on. It is direct apprehension unfolding in the present moment, followed spontaneously by a direct, hopefully appropriate action, if any action is called for or arises—which may not always be the case.

We are all capable of this kind of recognition in the present moment. We already engage in it when the circumstances spontaneously call it out of us. So why not in every moment? Why *not* recognize what is actually unfolding within you and around you moment by moment? That is mindfulness. It is that innate capacity for recognition of what is most salient, most important, most called for in this moment. You may discover that that capacity is profoundly trustworthy.

And we all already have it, or you might say, we all already are it. It is actually that very same capacity—simply seeing what is here to be seen, and then acting! That acting on the basis of what we apprehend, what we recognize, sometimes *looks* like doing nothing in that moment of awareness. But isn't, even if you don't do anything at all, including smile. Why? Because some shift has already come about within yourself. Why not acknowledge your innate capacity for recognition of things as they are, beyond how we label them and what we think about them, beyond their names and forms, drilling down to the essence of what is going on in the present moment, nonconceptually, before thinking sets in, or *underneath* whatever thoughts may be arising within us?

And why not then encourage that recognition to expand into other moments of our lives? Why not nurture that latent seed within ourselves? It is, after all, a form of intelligence. And it may in fact be our most endearing quality, and of all our human qualities, the capacity that might just be most critical to allowing us to evolve as a species at this moment in our development. Of course, some enterprising people will then start selling "kindfulness" bracelets or seminars, or whatever. But why buy or commodify something you already have? Something that is already an intrinsic part of who you are? Why not just befriend it? Why not use it as a kind of compass and live in accordance with its guidance?

Or to switch metaphors, why not see the world through the lens of direct apprehension, of recognition, and live in accordance with your own embodied values? Why not connect with others who care in the way that you care, and find new and imaginative ways to be in wiser relationship to our moments and to our opportunities to be of service to others and to ourselves? To transform society and establish not merely non-harming as a guiding principle in all our relationships, as in the Hippocratic Oath in medicine when it is lived up to, but also taking steps to heal the wounds of our social fabric, the wounds of racism, inequality, injustice, and poverty as best we can, mindfully wrestling with and hopefully transcending in moments of clarity our tribal impulses toward us-ing and them-ing, favoring those we identify as similar to ourselves, while demonizing, dehumanizing, abusing, or ignoring those who are different, and thus, ultimately and unwittingly, ourselves as well.

## Democracy 2.0—A Sorely Needed Upgrade via Mindfulness and Heartfulness

This book is about the realization of mindfulness not only in our own personal lives, but in the larger world we inhabit together. Thomas Jefferson once said: "Liberty is to the collective body what health is to the individual body. Without health no pleasure can be tasted by man; without liberty, no happiness can be enjoyed by society." He was right. At the same time, he was a slaveholder, denying liberty to other human beings in spite of his words in the Declaration of Independence that all (men) are created equal. So there is plenty of irony and contradiction here, and painful evidence of how slow the process of coming to a true democracy can be, and how challenging it is to break out of the box of one's own time and its multiple hard-to-see constraints that limit the evolution and realization of such an abstraction, however noble and worthy. Civilization's benefits always fall short of realization for some. The enslaved are always mindful of their enslavement. For them, it cannot be papered over with elevated rhetoric. They know the truth because they experience the oppression. Even ancient Athens, which gave us the concept of democracy, had slavery as an integral part of its social fabric. And when we speak of slavery, the polar opposite of being free, who could possibly imagine the suffering that it engendered and does to this day? The same could be said for the status of women, since the women of Athens were themselves excluded from the democratic process. For that matter, until less than one hundred years ago, a married woman in the United States did not have a legal existence apart from her husband.

This is one fundamental reason why democracy itself, and the liberation of all members of human society and the human family is usually a multigenerational evolutionary process, at present very much a work in progress with no guarantees of ultimate success, whatever that might be in a world where change is the only constant.

However, that cultural evolutionary process* is speeding up, along with time itself and the transformations that our sciences and technologies have wrought so far and will increasingly bring in the future, in our lifetime and in that of our children and grandchildren. So part of what is called for are enacted laws, democratically arrived at, that

---

* And perhaps, through epigenetic pathways, also biologically evolutionary as well.

protect the institutions of participation in the body politic, and the elemental sovereignty of all of its members, who constitute, if you will, the cells of the body politic for each country, and ultimately of the body politic of the planet.

Perhaps we could call this emergent possibility Democracy 2.0. It would be an "upgrade" that takes note of and prohibits all the various contradictions and machinations we have seen over the centuries that have sometimes, and even to this day* afforded outsized privilege to some members of society at the expense of others. This happens in a multiplicity of ways, from genocide and outright enslavement to endemic constraint through laws that favor the few—whether through inheritance, wealth, position, power, education, chicanery— over the many who have not had the benefit of such resources. The driver of this asymmetry is always ultimately greed, or hatred, or delusion, a protectionism of privilege, and a fundamental disregard for equal opportunity. Such elements curtail the right for *all* members of society (and the planet) to live life without undue and unfair constraints, be they legal, economic, social, or educational. Addressing this asymmetry will become even more important in society as many forms of human work/jobs are taken over by algorithms and robots.

Certainly there has been huge progress in standards of living, in health, and in personal wealth of ordinary citizens in first-world countries over the past two hundred years, and more recently, in almost all countries on the planet.† Yet the narrative of human liberty and equal justice for all that we teach to children and immigrants when they become citizens of the United States through the pledge of allegiance

---

* See, for example, Nancy MacLean, *Democracy in Chains: The Deep History of the Radial Right's Stealth Plan for America*, Viking, New York, 2017. Also Noam Chomsky, *Chomsky on Mis-Education*, Rowman & Littlefield, Lanham, MD, 2000.

† See Hans Rosling, *Factfulness: Ten Reasons We're Wrong About the World—And Why Things Are Better Than You Think*, Flatiron, New York, 2018; and Stephen Pinker, *Enlightenment Now: The Case for Reason, Science, Humanism, and Progress*, Viking, New York, 2018.

has not yet come to grips with the contradictions of our national origins in genocide and slavery, and the ways our laws and their sometimes rude and violent enforcement do indeed privilege the few in hugely asymmetric ways. Such asymmetries of privilege and power are even more flagrant in many other societies. The development of democracies within the sweep of the past several thousand years, from ancient Athens to now, has yet to face the roots of its own contradictions and the influence of powerful monied interests in subverting freedom and opportunity.

Now, I would say, it is about time for us as humans to catalyze an upgrade to a wisdom and compassion-based democracy, to assert that all beings have a fundamental right to life, liberty, and the pursuit of happiness—and to then inquire and investigate what true happiness might look like, and where it actually resides. Awareness of our own minds and desires has a huge role to play here, since ultimately, our minds and what we desire are at one and the same time the source of so much suffering and the only real possibility for liberation from that suffering, both for ourselves as individuals and for the world.

## The Power of Privilege and the Privilege of Power

As we all know, the Declaration of Independence, penned by Thomas Jefferson, speaks of "Life, Liberty, and the Pursuit of Happiness." But by the time the U.S. Constitution was enacted, the phrase "Pursuit of Happiness" was dropped in favor of "Property." Not so surprising, since the Constitution was a legal document, and all the signers were property owners (and white and men), whereas the Declaration of Independence was a revolutionary declaration of grievance, with no legal standing. In fact, that document signaled a turning away from the legal structures and strictures of the British Empire and an outright rejection of its domination of its colonies. These ironies are poignant evidence that the arc of democracy and freedom on this planet is just that, an evolutionary experiment unfolding over time, and vulnerable to being undermined in many different ways. So any absolutism around freedom or who has the power to decide things is limited and potentially blinding. In the end, democracy needs something else, transcending the exercise of raw power. It needs wisdom. And wisdom only comes from the realization that the pursuit of self-interest defined too narrowly engenders that very blindness, especially given that the notion of "self" is highly questionable, suspect even in us as human beings and citizens, never mind in terms of corporations and governments. For true happiness or well-being, in other words, to tap into Aristotle's *eudaemonia,* we need wakefulness, we need to learn to befriend our own essential nature as beings, as human beings. This is the domain of the non-dual, underneath thinking, beyond thinking, the realm of awareness itself (see Book 2, *Falling Awake: How to Practice Mindfulness in Everyday Life*).

## The Practice of Non-Doing

Non-doing, an essential element of the cultivation of mindfulness, almost sounds un-American, so much are we a culture of enterprising doers and go-getters. But the non-doing/being option through which we can understand and ground all our doing, individual and collective, is becoming increasingly attractive to us as Americans. It is an invitation to be true to the promise of what an enlightened democratic society might be at this point in time, and to equally beware of the impulses of greed, hatred, and delusion—especially when undergirded and abetted by unjust laws—that could undermine it or subvert it altogether, an increasingly scary specter in this digital age. As the U.S. Air Force motto has it: Eternal vigilance is the price of freedom. If the Air Force only knew how true that motto is. But the vigilance has to come out of a clear mind and a wise heart, and be grounded in an ethical and moral soil. Otherwise that freedom can all-too-easily become part of the newspeak of George Orwell's dystopic *1984*. It can also give rise to what we saw unfold in the White House in 2018 in perhaps increasingly more grotesque, overt, and disturbingly dangerous ways than in the past, but which indeed, has always been a tendency within human society that periodically comes into ascendency, takes root, and takes over. And when it does, invariably a lot of people die. A lot of people, even children, are imprisoned unjustly. And love and compassion seemingly die with it.

Only that never happens entirely. That is another limited narrative we can tell ourselves and feel authenticated in in the short run, depending on our beliefs and allegiances. Human kindness and caring cannot die. Awareness and wisdom cannot die. They are in our DNA, often emerging under even the harshest and most nightmarish conditions. Each one of us is capable of great love as well as, unfortunately, great harm to others and to ourselves, both by comission and omission. Why not nurture the love? Why not nurture wisdom? Why not incline our minds and hearts in this direction? After all, it is where real freedom and happiness lie.

## A Larger Vision of Self and Self-Interest

Let's nurture life as best we can by expanding our definition of "self-interest" and looking deeply into what we even mean by self, and by "me" and "mine," by "us" and "them" and what happens to "us" when we fall into the trap of reflexive emotional distancing and dehumanizing. We might inquire similarly about true well-being and happiness if we manage to write ourselves restraining orders in this regard at key moments, gentle reminders that we do not have to reflexively go this route of us-ing and them-ing on the personal level or at the level of the body politic.

## Shaping the Future by Showing Up in This Moment

And, while we are at it, let's marvel at our potential role in what is yet to come, and contribute to it each in our own way by taking care of this moment fully. When we do, the next moment is already profoundly different, because we chose to show up fully in this one. This is how we shape the future, how we bring about a wiser and kinder future—by taking care of and responding to the *present* we have now with our full presence and multiple intelligences, in other words, mindfully, in awareness.

This book invites you to trust your own creativity and heritage in that regard, whatever country or culture you belong to or view you identify with. Through the ongoing *cultivation* of mindfulness and heartfulness, we contribute, each in our own small but hardly insignificant way, to a multidimensional interconnected lattice-structure in which we can be nodes of embodied wisdom that can incrementally heal and transform our world. Embodied wisdom emerges in how we take care of and interact with our children and grandchildren in the moment rather than in the abstract. It manifests in the world we bequeath to them. It resides within the work we do, in our relationships, in our willingness to affirm what we most value and embody it in how we carry ourselves in our actions and in our choices. It appears when we are willing to sit down and listen wholeheartedly to others who may see things very differently from how we see things, when we listen deeply to nature, including to our own true nature, and to the universe itself. In a word, embodied wisdom is alive and well when we are fully alive and well, when we manage from moment to moment and from day to day to recognize and then put out the welcome mat for what is—including the full catastrophe of the human condition—and then tend it wisely. When we do, the cultivation of mindfulness winds up somehow, mysteriously, connecting us to life itself in deep ways we might not have imagined possible and thus, winds up ultimately being of benefit to all.

## Looking Back to See Ahead

As you will see from the examples I draw from, especially in Part 1, the bulk of the material in this book was first written between 2002 and 2004, as the last two parts of the original *Coming to Our Senses*. There, I attempted to expand the scope of the practice of mindfulness and its intrinsically orthogonal orientation to include "the body politic," in other words, to extend its healing potential to society as a whole—to the way the United States of America actually behaves at home and in the world as opposed to its rhetoric—as well as to some of the critical challenges our species was beginning to realize it was facing at that time, and is facing even more so now, in this moment.

This book is an optimistic attempt to make the case that it is imperative for us as human beings to bring the lens and cultivation of mindfulness* to the larger world and to the planet as a whole. In doing so, we might have a much better framework for accurately diagnosing and then appropriately treating the ills of our society, both in terms of outright disease and the underlying and pervasive dis-ease (see Book 1, Part 2) it is suffering from. The outright disease element would include the incontrovertible evidence that the activity of our species has managed to give the planet a fever that has the potential to make life infinitely harder for almost everybody in the next few generations, and perhaps even unlivable, without some radical if not miraculous planet-wide social, technological, and governmental innovations of major proportions, coupled with reining in our seemingly endless intoxication with growth.

But the biggest learning, growing, healing, and transformation will not come out of technology or government. It can only come from our capacity as human beings—all of us—to wake up to our predicament and to our potential for realization: realization of our circumstances and of both the inner as well as the outer resources available to us as a species to minimize what is unhealthy and often greed-driven for something healthier and more compassionate. And out of that realization, to mobilize those resources, each and every one of

---

* that we saw in Book 3 can be instrumental in reclaiming, healing, and transforming our personal lives

us, in the service of healing rather than harming. We need to address head-on, with the full range of our multiple intelligences—somatic, intuitive, conceptual, emotional, social, global—what our precocious species has objectively wrought since the dawn of the Industrial Revolution, only a dozen human generations ago—the shadow side as well as the beauty.

*

As you will see, I made the deliberate choice for the current volume not to rewrite this material in its entirety and deploy more contemporaneous examples. Instead, I lightly tweaked and added to the text here and there to bring certain elements up to date. Most of the examples are by now historical. And yet not! We keep seeing the same themes and tendencies played out over and over again today that were apparent in the early 2000s, when it was written, and long before that. How we treat the world in this moment depends in large measure, as it always has, on the lenses we use to apprehend it, and the attributions we make to comprehend it. We are seeing divisiveness played out as never before, and yet, as always before. The technology may be faster and more pervasive, since we have globally networked supercomputers in our pockets and handbags, but the basic elements of our species' struggle remain the same.

I hope you will be able to see through the lenses of these pages the world as it is now, and realize in your own way what it would take to live fully the life that is yours to live in the climate (all puns intended) we find ourselves in now—and what it would take to insure the same for everybody else. If we approach the dis-ease of the human condition from a medical perspective—drawing on what medicine and science have learned (see Book 3) about the mind/body connection, neuroplasticity, epigenetics, telomeres and cellular aging, and indeed, about mindfulness, health, and well-being, public health, and the environment over the past forty years, we may just have a chance to diagnose our condition with much greater accuracy than in the past. And as a consequence, to find and have the motivation and stamina to implement an appropriate course of treatment for the magnitude of what ails us. In the process, we have the opportunity to uncover, discover, and recover our intrinsic wholeness and original beauty as human beings. That is not only satisfying—it gives rise to deep insight, and thus, to real power.

*

As essential "cells" of the body politic and of the flowering of life on this planet, each one of us counts, and our efforts to cultivate and embody mindfulness (and thus heartfulness and kindfulness) in our own lives and in our richly diverse relationships may be *the* critical element—and may in the end make *the* critical difference—in how things unfold in the coming moments, years, and generations.

There is cause for optimism. As my late father-in-law, the historian, teacher, and civil rights and peace activist, Howard Zinn put it:

We don't have to engage in grand heroic actions to participate in the process of change. Small acts, when multiplied by millions of people, can transform the world. To be hopeful in bad times is not just foolishly romantic. It is based on the fact that human history is a history not only of cruelty, but also of compassion, sacrifice, courage, kindness. What we choose to emphasize in this complex history will determine our lives. If we see only the worst, it destroys our capacity to do something. If we remember those times and places—and there are so many—where people have behaved magnificently, this gives us the energy to act, and at least the possibility of sending this spinning top of a world in a different direction.

And if we do act, in however small a way, we don't have to wait for some grand utopian future. The future is an infinite succession of presents, and to live *now* as we think human beings should live, in defiance of all that is bad around us, is itself a marvelous victory.*

\*

May your mindfulness practice continue to grow and flower and nourish your life and health and work and calling in this world from moment to moment and from day to day. May the beauty of the world hold you during the best of times and the worst of times, and remind you of who you really really really really are and what is most important to keep alive and flourishing while you have the chance.

May you walk in beauty, as the Navaho people say, and may you realize that you already do—and that you always have. And may you tend what needs tending in the world along the way, with tenderness.

Jon Kabat-Zinn
Northampton, MA
October 26, 2018

---

\* H. Zinn, *You Can't Be Neutral on a Moving Train: A Personal History of Our Times*, Beacon Press, Boston, 1994, 2002. See also the Zinn Education Project (ZEP): https://www.zinnedproject.org/.

# PART 1

# HEALING THE BODY POLITIC

# HEALING THE BODY POLITIC

*Power at its best is love implementing the demands of justice, and
justice at its best is power correcting everything that stands against
love.*

### MARTIN LUTHER KING

Everything that we have touched on so far in our explorations of
mindfulness on the personal level in the first three books in this series
applies equally well to our behavior in the world as a country and as
a species. Look at any event going on today. Do we actually know
what is really happening? Or are we merely forming opinions based
on trusting or mistrusting specific news outlets, based on reflexive
preferences that have us aligning ourselves with some narratives and
rejecting others out-of-hand, caught up in "us-ing" and "them-ing,"
liking and disliking, wanting or fearing certain things, caught in the
surface appearance of things, or imagining what is going on beneath
the surface but without, when you come right down to it, actually
knowing?

Here is the challenge: Can we apply the non-dual lens of mindful awareness to what is going on in the world and to our interface
with it as an integral unit (cell) of the body politic that is our society
and our country, whichever country you reside in or identify with?
For instance, can we bring mindfulness to what presents itself to our

senses and mobilize our capacity for discernment and not-knowing when it comes to "the news"? Can we be aware of those events, big and little, that have varying degrees of impact sooner or later on our private and personal lives, but which are often very much removed from our direct experience and what is actually occurring in our daily lives—that is, until they are not? And then, when they are not, can we bring awareness to those moments when, all of a sudden, we find ourselves swept up and powerfully affected directly or indirectly by forces we have not fully understood, whether they be primarily economic, social, political, geopolitical, military, environmental, medical, or some complex combination of these such as global warming, or the changing mores around gender, or the very real challenges of mass migrations of peoples fleeing from the suffering of war or famine or the like? These forces are inevitably much larger than we are. They perturb the comfort of our personal concerns, traditions, and cultures. That can be painful and fear-inducing. Yet those very same forces also have the potential, if we don't resist them out of that impulse to fall into fear, to catapult us into a larger perspective because far more fundamental human issues are at stake.

So in the end, the challenge is whether or not we can be orthogonal.* Is it possible for us to be more openhearted, more inclusive, without it threatening our own sense of well-being and safety too much? Is it possible for us to *embody* compassion? Can we embody wisdom in how we respond to change and uncertainty and possible threats to our sense of who we are as individuals and as a country or a species? Can we be wise? These are our challenges today when it comes to the outer world, as they are with the interior world of our own minds and hearts. Outer and inner being reflections of each other affords us infinite opportunities for shaping our relationship with both, and in turn, being shaped by them. Perhaps here too, as a society, there is every possibility to greet ourselves arriving at our own door and to

---

* See Book 3, Part 1.

love again the stranger who was ourself, in the words of Derek Walcott's poem *Love After Love* that took us to the close of Book 3.

We only need to hark back to the old lady/young lady figure, or the Kanizsa triangle in Book 1 to remind ourselves that we can easily see certain aspects of things and not others, or believe strongly in the reality of something that may be more an illusion than an actuality. And those are simple examples compared to the fluxing complexity of issues and situations we face in our lives every day, to say nothing of those that are faced by our country and the world. All of us, especially if we do not pay sufficient attention to *how* we see and *how* we know, wind up all too often mis-perceiving complex situations and getting myopically attached to an incomplete or partial view. When we do, we may be excluding out of hand other dimensions of whatever the issue is that need to be recognized as perhaps having some degree of validity that we simply don't want to see. This foxholing mentality, this at least partially blind attachment to an interpretation of events that may only be true to a degree, if it is true at all, creates enmity and suffering—for ourselves and for others. Might not our institutions and our politics become healthier and wiser if we all engaged even a little bit in expanding the field of our awareness inwardly and outwardly to entertain the possible validity, at least to a degree, of ways of knowing, seeing, and being that may be profoundly different from our own?

Whatever opinions you hold or don't hold, whether they be political, religious, economic, cultural, historical, social, or just positions you take within your family about the various issues that come up daily, you might want to consider for a moment those who hold a diametrically opposite opinion. Are they all completely deluded? Are they all "bad people"? Might there not be a tendency in yourself to dehumanize them, to stereotype them, even to demonize them? Do you find yourself generalizing about a certain "them" and making sweeping statements about them and "their" character or intelligence or even their humanity? If we start paying attention in this way to the activity of our own minds, recognizing our thoughts as just thoughts, our opinions as just opinions, and our emotions as emotions, we may rapidly discover that this generalizing and lumping into fixed categories can happen even with the people we live with and love the most. That is why family is usually such a wonderful, as well as sometimes maddening, laboratory for honing greater awareness, compassion, and wisdom, and for actually implementing and embodying them moment by moment in our everyday lives. For when we find ourselves clinging strongly to the certainty that we are right and others are wrong, even if it is true to a large degree and the stakes are very very high (or at least we think they are and are sorely attached to our view of it), then our very lenses of perception can become distorted, and we risk falling into delusion and doing some degree of violence to the actuality of the situation and to the relationships we are in, far beyond the "objective" validity and merit of one position or another. When I examine my own mind, I have to recognize that I am subject to all those tendencies every day and have to watch out for them so as to not become majorly deluded. I imagine I am not unique in that regard.

If there is even a bit of that going on—and the same is, in all likelihood, going on for those who hold opinions opposite to your own, when they think about you and those who see things "your way"—is this situation even remotely likely to capture what is really going on, and the potential for the recognition of at least some common ground and shared interests and a greater truth? Or has the way we are seeing and thinking so polarized the situation or topic or issue, whatever issue it is, and so blinded us that it is no longer really possible to see and know things as they actually are? Or even to remember that we really don't know, and that there is huge creative and potentially healing power in that not knowing. It is not ignorance nor is it ignorant. It is compassionate. It is wise. That knowing that we don't know is more powerful, and more healing than building walls out of fear, or pointing fingers, or going to war on pretext, or us-ing and them-ing endlessly.

Knowing that we don't know, or that we usually only know something to a degree, can provide huge openings and orthogonal emergences to arise in our minds and hearts that would not be otherwise possible. Remember what the Korean Zen Master, Soen Sa Nim (Books 1 and 3), would do with anyone who was clinging to any position. "If you say this is a stick, or a watch, or a table, a good situation, or a bad situation, or the truth, I will hit you thirty times [metaphorically—he didn't really hit anybody]. And if you say this is not a stick, or a watch, or a table, a good situation, or a bad situation, or the truth, I will hit you thirty times. What can you do?"

Remember, he was actually reminding us to wake up from this-or-that, black-or-white, good-or-bad, us-or-them thinking. It was an act of compassion to put us in this quandary, or to point out that we actually get there all the time on our very own.

Yes, what can you do? What can we do? And in the end, what about calling a spade a spade? What about genocide, murder, exploitation, corporate crimes, political corruption, institutionalized patterns of deceit (online and off), structural racism, and injustice? Yes, of course we can, and sometimes, morally, we *must* stand up and call a spade a spade when you or I actually *know* it is a spade. But if you know it, and you are really seeing it clearly and not merely clinging to your idea of "spade," then you will see instantly that calling it a spade may not be the only or the most important thing, especially if that is all you do. There may be something more appropriate to the situation than putting forth a concept or a label, however important standing up and accurately naming what is happening is, and it is extremely important. There may also be a compelling necessity to act, and act wisely, to find an embodied way through which you can be in relationship with what is unfolding with integrity and dignity, something you can actually *do* that goes beyond merely naming or calling names, or agreeing with others who are doing the same.

If it were literally a spade, then maybe picking it up and beginning to dig and getting others to work alongside you might be appropriate. Acting to embody our understanding of what is going on in any moment may be the best we can do in any moment, and would approach wisdom incrementally if we were willing to learn from the consequences of our actions. Everything else may devolve rapidly into empty talk. The politician running for office says it is a spade, and something has to be done about it. Once in office, why is it that his or her view of its reality and importance can alter so radically and so rapidly? Metaphorically speaking, is it still a spade, or was it just a spade for convenience in that moment, as a stepping-stone to something else?

Paraphrasing Bertrand Russell, human beings have learned to fly in the air and descend underneath the sea. But we haven't yet learned to live on the land. The last frontier for us is not the oceans, nor outer space, as interesting and enticing as they may be. The last and most important and most urgent frontier for us is the human mind and the human heart. It is knowing ourselves, and most importantly, from the inside! The last frontier is really consciousness itself. It is the coming together of everything we know, of all the wisdom traditions of all the peoples of this planet, including all our different ways of knowing, through science, through the arts, through native traditions, through meditative inquiry, through embodied mindfulness practices. This is the challenge of our era and of our species, now that we are so networked together throughout the world in so many ways, so that what happens in Helsinki, or Moscow, or in tweets from the White House, what happens in Brussels or Baghdad or Kuala Lumpur, or in Mexico City or New York or Washington, or Kabul, or Beijing or anywhere else can wind up deeply affecting people's lives the next day or the next month virtually anywhere and even everywhere else in the world. And that is to say nothing of the dissipative pressures continually threatening democracy itself, real inclusivity, and equal justice under the law, so that all the "cells" of the body politic can benefit from an equal "blood supply." It is the exact opposite of burying our heads in the sand and preoccupying ourselves with our own narrowly defined self-interest and with maximizing our own safety or happiness or gain. Rather, our entire exploration of mindfulness and the possibilities of healing our lives and the world is offering us a way to look around at the forest from time to time and know it directly in its fullness rather than being so caught up in minute preoccupations with individual trees and branches, as important as that level of understanding may be. It is reminding us that without the distorting lenses of narrowly conceived and unexamined thoughts and opinions, usually driven by varying degrees of fear, greed, hatred, and delusion, and of course, by an endemic tribalism, the age-old instinct to fall into us-ing and them-ing, incubated and inflamed in this era by talk radio and social networks, including malevolent internet entities which may be bots, and pervasive tendencies on all sides to disregard realistic evidence—is a huge and blinding trap, preventing us from seeing new openings and possibilities.

Not to say that there is not a place for opinions and strongly held views. Only that the more those views take into account the inter-embeddedness of things on the micro and macro levels, the better our ability to interface with the world and with our work and with our longing and our calling in ways that will contribute to greater wisdom and harmony, as opposed to greater strife and misery and insecurity.

Now, more than ever before, on virtually all fronts, we have a priceless opportunity and the wherewithal, both individually and collectively, not to get caught up and blinded by our destructive emotions and our unexamined self-centeredness, but rather to come to our senses, both literally and metaphorically. In doing so, perhaps we will wake up to and recognize the dis-ease that has become increasingly a chronic condition of our world and species over the past ten thousand years of human history, and take practical steps to envision and nurture new possibilities for balance and harmony in how we conduct our lives as individuals and our interactions as nations, ways that recognize and strive to minimize our own destructive tendencies and sheer nastiness at times, mind states that only feed dis-ease and alienation, inwardly and outwardly, and instead maximize our capacity for mobilizing and embodying wisdom and compassion in the choices we make from moment to moment about how we need to be living, and what we might be doing with our creative energies to heal the body politic.

*

Throughout these four volumes, we have been exploring the metaphors of disease and dis-ease in attempting to define and understand, from many different angles, the deep nature of our disquietude as human beings, and why so much of the time we feel so out of joint, so much in need of something we sense is missing in order to feel complete, even though, materially and in terms of education and many other factors, we are far better off in developed countries and for that matter, in the majority of what used to be called "developing" countries, than the vast majority of human beings ever were in any generations preceding ours.* If a relatively high standard of living, material wealth and abundance, and even better health and health care than ever before in history are not sufficient for us to be happy, contented, and inwardly at peace, what might still be missing? And what would it take for us to appreciate who we are and what we already have? And what is our discontent telling us about ourselves as a country, as a world, and as a species that we might benefit from knowing? How might we cease being strangers to ourselves and come home to who we actually are in our fullness? How might we know and embody our true nature and our true potential as human beings?

Looking inwardly for a moment, we might ask ourselves, what *would* it take for us as individuals within the body politic to *feel* whole and happy right now, given that in actuality, as we have seen over and

---

* See Hans Rosling, *Factfulness: Ten Reasons We're Wrong About the World—And Why Things Are Better Than You Think,* Flatiron, New York, 2018; also Steven Pinker: *Enlightenment Now: The Case for Reason, Science, Humanism, and Progress,* Viking, New York, 2018.

over again through our cultivation of mindfulness, we *are* already undeniably whole and complete in this very moment. One thing that it might take is to expand out beyond living so much of the time in our heads and caught up in our thoughts and desires and the turbulence of our reactive emotions and addictions, whether it be to food (the obesity epidemic) or to numbing our pain (the opioid epidemic), or to something else. In the end, we seem to be imprisoned by our own endless and often desperate attempts to arrange external circumstances, causes, and conditions so that—we always hope—they will bring about a better situation in which we will finally be able to extinguish the pain and be happy and at peace.

Underneath even that, we might recognize our habitual, seductive, but ultimately misplaced preoccupation with a remarkably persistent but at the same time amazingly ungraspable sense of a solid, enduring, unchanging personal self. That elusive solid-self feeling, when examined through the lens of mindfulness, is easily seen to be something of an illusion. I think we all know this deep down in our hearts. Yet that sense of a permanent solid self and the self-centeredness that accompanies it seems to continually mesmerize us and drive us here and there in pursuit of its seemingly endless needs and wants. When we wake up for even brief moments to the mystery of who we are, that self-construct is seen to be so much smaller than the full extent of our being. This is as true for the country and for the world as it is for us as individuals.

In the end, these insights and the openings that can accompany them stem from cultivating greater moment-to-moment intimacy and familiarity with our own minds and bodies, and from realizing the interconnectedness of things beyond our perceptions of them being separate and disconnected, and beyond our delusion-generating attachment to their being under our tight control and for our own narrow benefit.

Our wholeness and interdependence can actually be verified here and now, in any and every moment through waking up and realizing that, in the deepest of ways, we and the world we inhabit are not two. As we have seen, there are any number of ways to cultivate and nurture this wakefulness through the systematic practice of mindfulness. All apply equally well in taking on a more universal awareness of and responsibility for the health of the body politic in any and every sense of it.

*

Through the practice of mindfulness, of looking deeply into ourselves, we have been cultivating greater familiarity and intimacy with what might possibly be the ultimate, root causes of our disquietude and our suffering, the dynamics of greed, hatred, and unawareness as mind states, and how many different ways they have of manifesting in the world. Perhaps we have come to see or sense to some extent how we might, each one of us in our own way, more effectively contribute to reducing suffering, mitigating suffering, and transcending suffering—our own and that of others—and to extinguishing the human *causes* of that suffering at their root, inwardly and outwardly, wherever possible.

Perhaps it may have also dawned on us that we cannot be completely healthy or at peace in our own private lives inhabiting a world that itself is diseased and so much not at peace, in which so much of the suffering is inflicted by human beings upon one another, directly and indirectly, and upon the Earth, primarily as a consequence of our lack of understanding of interconnectedness and often, it seems, a lack of caring even when we "know better." Of course, this is endemically human behavior, but it too can be worked with if we are willing to do a certain kind of inner work as individuals and as a society. Even endemic small-mindedness is amenable to change if we come to see the potential value in learning to live and act differently, with a greater awareness of the interdependency and inter-embeddedness of self and of other and of the true needs and true nature of both self and other, in other words, if we can learn to recognize the distorting lenses of our own greed, fear, hatred, and unawareness when they arise, and not let them obscure deeper and healthier elements of who and what we are. All this comes from being willing to visit and hold our own pain and suffering, as individuals, as a nation, and as a species, with awareness, compassion, and some degree of non-reactivity, letting them speak to us and reveal new dimensions of interconnectedness that increase our understanding of those root causes of suffering and compel us to extend our empathy out beyond only those people we are closest to. It means that people everywhere have to have their basic needs met and be free from exploitation, injustice, and degradation at the hands of others. In other words, it means that all people everywhere have to have their basic human rights protected. As we know, this is sadly not the case for vast numbers of human beings on the planet at this time, in our own country and throughout the world.

It is not inappropriate to use the metaphor of an autoimmune disease to describe the effect of our species on the planet, and even on our own health and well-being as a species. Another way to put it is that we humans somehow keep getting in our own way. We keep tripping over obstacles we unwittingly throw in our own path, in spite of all our cleverness. Throughout these four volumes, I have been suggesting that what we have learned in medicine in the past forty years about the mind/body connection and the potential healing power of mindfulness/heartfulness can have profound applications in the way we understand and deal with the overwhelming dis-ease from which the greater body of our nation and the greater body of this one world are suffering. The symptoms of this dis-ease are writ large in our newspapers, cable news, talk radio, and newsfeeds every single day in breathtaking ways that defy imagination and even at times call our basic sanity into question.

As with every other aspect of this exploration we have undertaken— of mindfulness as a meditation practice and as a way of being—the aim in examining the domain of the body politic in relationship to mindfulness is not to change opinions, our own or others', nor to confirm them. Cultivating greater mindfulness in our lives does not imply that we would fall into one set of ideological views and opinions or another, however appealing that might be at times. Rather, it offers us the opportunity to see things freshly, for ourselves, with eyes of wholeness, moment by moment. What mindfulness can do for us is to *reveal* our opinions, and all opinions, *as opinions*. With that kind of recognition, we will know them for what they are and perhaps not be so caught by them and blinded by them, whatever their content, even when we sometimes adopt particular positions quite consciously and hold them strongly and with conviction, and act on them. The invitation of mindfulness in this regard is to look into the mirror of your own mind, apprehend your own strong attachments, and explore unrecognized possibilities for healing and inquiry and perhaps for an expansion of the way we see things, rather than merely falling into some kind of reflexive partisan agreement or disagreement on specific issues. This way of being in relationship with experience, with reality as it is, is thus an invitation to change lenses altogether, to experiment with a rotation in consciousness that may be as large as the world itself, or, often at the very same time, as close as this moment and this breath, in this body, within this mind and this heart that you and I and all of us bring to the nowscape (Book 2, Part 1). This is the essence and the gift of mindfulness as a formal meditation practice and as a way of being, a way of living.

The aim here is also to remind us that there is nothing passive about awareness. Our state of mind in any moment and everything that flows from it affects the world. When our doing comes out of being, out of awareness, it is likely to be a wiser, freer, more imaginative, more creative, and a more caring doing, a doing that can itself catalyze greater wisdom and compassion and healing in the world and in your own heart. The intentional engagement in mindfulness within various strata of society, and within the body politic, even in the tiniest of ways, has the potential, because we are all cells of the one body of the world, to lead to a true flowering, a veritable renaissance of human creativity and potential, an expression of our profound intrinsic health as a species, and as a world. It is already happening in many different domains, in tiny ways that aren't so tiny. The renaissance is already here.

The suggestion that the world might benefit from all of us taking greater responsibility for its well-being and bringing greater mindfulness to the body politic is not meant to be a prescription for a particular treatment to fix a particular problem, or even to describe the problems we are facing in any detail and attribute blame to particular parties, individuals, customs, or ways of thinking, much as there may be a reflexive impulse to do so at particular moments. Rather, it is meant to be impressionistic, just as an impressionist painting reveals itself in its fullness and depth only when you stand back at a certain distance and take in the whole of it and don't get too preoccupied with the individual dabs of paint. It is also meant to be lovingly provocative, an invitation for all of us to take a fresh look at and challenge our most cherished assumptions, attachments, fears, and perhaps our unexamined viewpoints and lenses, a call for all of us to begin paying attention in new ways. It is also a call for us to examine more carefully the very ways in which we perceive or know anything, or think we perceive and know something. It is an invitation to engage in mindfully investigating the very process by which we form opinions and then make a strong link between our identity (who we think we are and who we identify with) and those very opinions.

It is also an invitation to begin imagining new metaphors for understanding ourselves and our place in the world, and for honoring the very real complexities of the real world without losing sight of the fact that the minds of human beings have in large measure created—you could say fabricated and proliferated—many of the problems we now face as a country and as a species, and that, like everything else, they are not as permanent, enduring, or as real as our minds make them out to be. This insight alone may afford us new and imaginative ways of dealing with what often seem like intractable situations and enmities. It may be worth reminding ourselves here of two famous comments from Albert Einstein. In the first, he said, "Reality is merely an illusion, albeit a very persistent one." In the second, he said, "The problems that exist in the world today cannot be solved by the level of thinking that created them." Both of these observations are worth keeping in mind as we cultivate mindfulness in full face of the full catastrophe of the human condition.

We might say that the human mind has fabricated the very notion of the "real world" along with the constraints we usually impose on ourselves in thinking about it and about what might even be possible in the same way it constructs a reified notion of a permanent self. If we examine and become acutely aware of how our minds perceive, apprehend, and conceive of both ourselves and what we call the world, then many of those self-imposed, illusory constraints may dissolve as we find new ways to act based on this rotation in consciousness.

The specifics will come out of our ongoing practice in the conduct of our day-to-day lives. The mentality that merely wants to fix things and set everything straight by imposing some special "solution" or reform that we believe in very strongly is not likely to be entirely helpful by itself, however important such efforts may be. A more global healing of our ways of seeing and being is also needed. This requires a broad-based rotation in consciousness on the part of large numbers of people, all of us, really, and a willingness to recognize things as they are and work with them in imaginative orthogonal ways, making use of all the vast resources and expertise available to us inwardly and outwardly. Rather than hoping for some special "savior" in the form of a charismatic leader who will "do it for us" or "show us the way," perhaps we have reached the point in our evolution as a species where we humans will need to move beyond a history governed by heroic and galvanizing personalities, no matter how larger-than-life they may be, on the good side or the nefarious side, and find ways to let the responsibility and the leadership be more distributive and cooperative, just as the heart and the liver and the brain do not fight among themselves to dominate the organism, but work together for the seamless well-being of the whole, as do the trillions of individual cells which together comprise a healthy human body.

Faced with an underlying root diagnosis of *dukkha* in all its various meanings and connotations (see Book 1), which we might alternatively call "world stress," and with an understanding of some of the underlying causes for *dukkha*, if there is a prescription here for a treatment for our current situation as a species, it is a generic one: that, strange as it may sound, whoever is touched by the dilemma we find ourselves facing as a species and as a society engage in the cultivation of greater mindfulness, as a practice and as a way of being; that we bring mindfulness gracefully and gently to every aspect of our lives and work, without knowing or having to know what will come of it, whoever we are, whatever our work and our calling; and that we practice it and embody it as best we can, individually and collectively, as if our lives and our very world depended on it.

For how we choose to live and to act from moment to moment influences the world in small ways that may be disproportionately beneficial, especially if the motivation our choices come out of is wholesome and ethical and the actions themselves wise and compassionate. In this way, the healing of the body politic can evolve without rigid control or direction, through the independent and interdependent agency and efforts of many different people and institutions, with many different and rich perspectives, aims, and interests, but with a common and potentially unifying interest as well, that of the greater well-being of the world. At its best, this is what politics both furthers and protects.

Of course, not everyone is going to take up the practice of mindfulness, either in the near term or the long term. But bit by bit, as has been happening for years, through many different improbable or even heretofore unimaginable avenues, those who are choosing this path to greater sanity and wisdom are growing, both in number and in potential influence. In the next few generations, say in the next several hundred years, as well as for us in this very moment, we have a remarkable opportunity—as individual human beings, as nations, and as a species—to realize the full potential of our creativity and our ability to see clearly, and put them to work in the service of wholeness, healing, and inclusivity. We can put them to work for what we all claim we most desire and would give us the greatest chance for feeling secure and happy: justice, compassion, fairness, freedom from oppression, equal opportunities for living fully and well, and thus, peace, goodwill, and love—and not just for ourselves or those with whom we most closely identify, but for all human beings, and for all sentient beings, with whom we are inextricably linked in so many life-giving and life-sustaining ways.

We are sitting atop a unique moment in history unfolding, a major tipping point. Whether it is evolutionary or revolutionary or both, this time we are in provides singular opportunities that can be seized and made use of with every breath. There is only one way to do that. It is to embody in our lives as they are unfolding here and now, our deepest values and our understanding of what is most important—and share it with each other, trusting that such embodied actions, on even the smallest of scales, will entrain the world into greater wisdom and health and sanity.

That is one hell of a practice. But again, for each one of us, what else is there worth doing with our one wild and precious life?

## "I Read the News Today, Oh Boy"

I flip on the TV news, or pick up a newspaper and start reading, or these days, on occasion check it on my phone. What a perplexing tangle of different forces at play in the world. The mind and the heart are instantly bombarded with a cacophony of suffering and endless analyses and opinions about it taking a multiplicity of forms and perspectives. How are we, who are not experts in international affairs or politics or economics or social policy or criminal justice, or even of history, to grasp the enormity and the minutiae of what is actually going on and the ultimate significance of any of it? It feels like a huge cascading torrent, this day's recounting of what happened, who said what, who did what, who knew what when and who didn't, who went where, who responded to what and how they responded. There was such a recounting yesterday. There will be another one tomorrow. And none of it, mind you, is exactly what happened. They are *stories* about what happened, constrained by all sorts of parameters, some of which we know, some of which we may have no inkling of, much of it "spun" one way or another by pundits and by political protagonists aiming to achieve or prevent one effect or another. The boundary between fact and opinion is becoming blurrier and blurrier, and the need for clarity and discernment in taking it in more and more essential—if we choose to take it in at all, given its overall toxicity. In fact, there are so many mutually exclusive narratives that pass for "the news" that we are forced to live in bubbles of relative misinformation and slant, and it is often merely a choice between what bubble you want to be affiliated with and mesmerized by, although some bubbles seem to care at least in principle much more deeply for the First Amendment and some modicum of accuracy and veracity than others. One day we witness enforced separation of children from their families in the land of the free and the home of the brave. Unconscionable, yet it became a reality. We do that. But the fact is that throughout our history, horrible things have been done and condoned by our government, including by the Supreme Court. Our history is not exactly the triumphalist narrative we were fed in our history books in school. Regular people have always spoken out against injustice in protest, often at great risk to themselves. But *that* history has not been taught in our schools until relatively recently.*

We can glean a lot by taking in the news, however it comes to us, through the lens of our own discernment and wisdom. Whether we know it or not, we are continually building our own images and opinions of the world and what is going on out of this never-ending stream of partial information to which we can easily become addicted, even as we are perhaps becoming exasperated and outraged by particular emergences, the particulars depending, of course, on who you are and what you care about or are even open to hearing or cannot escape admitting. Our eyes flitting over the newspaper or down the screen in your hand fill the mind with random details as much as with coherent stories or analysis, out of which grow our own thoughts, reactive emotions, and whatever opinions we form, all of which tend to proliferate endlessly. Watching the news on TV or listening to it on the radio does much the same. After a while, however we take it in, it becomes a steady diet, and a poor one. For most of the news is a

---

* See, for instance, H. Zinn and A. Arnove, *Voices of a People's History of the United States: 10th Anniversary Edition,* Seven Stories Press, New York, 2004, 2009. Also, the American history curricula provided on the Zinn Education Project (ZEP) website: https://www.zinnedproject.org.

recounting of dukkha in its infinite forms. There is precious little to lift the spirits.

Actually, there is a great deal to lift the spirits, but you have to search it out and listen carefully for it.

The news is different every day, yet there is a certain sameness to it over days, weeks, months, and even years...it's just the news. In total, it is hard to know what to make of it, how to hold it, and how to respond to it. It is so graphic, and at the same time, so abstract and impersonal—at least, until it becomes horribly personal. It is hard to know what to think, what is actually happening, and whose stories to believe. At least I find it hard. Very hard. Beyond the bare-bones facts—and even those are usually grossly and even grotesquely contested in this and most likely every era—perhaps it is impossible.

What is more, on one level or another, subtle or not so subtle, the endless stream of news we are immersed in, including in many instances outright hacking from various sources intent on sowing misinformation to tilt and disrupt the social order, stimulates thinking in us, lots of thinking. We need to become much more mindful of that fact and its unrecognized effects on our emotions and our views and tacit assumptions. Through cultivating mindfulness, we can readily see that our thinking, even at its best, is only one of a multiplicity of human intelligences (including somatic, emotional, cognitive, intuitive, interpersonal, societal) and that it is best held in awareness and recognized *as thinking* rather than being perceived as actual fact. In awareness, we can catch ourselves forming opinions, sometimes very strong opinions, coupled with strong emotions, when taking in the news we are immersed in. We can recognize what is happening in that very moment or soon after. This can be a way to intentionally maintain both clarity and equanimity in the face of the never-ending onslaught, especially in those moments when we are faced with major crises of conscience and morality that can shake us to our very foundation, like when children and their teachers are killed in school shootings, an unimaginable event that has become heartrendingly common, and diagnostic of something deeply amiss in our society.

On a daily basis, the news stream is likely to stimulate huge anxiety and insecurity in us, as well as anger and resentment. The body contracts with tension that is not easy to release on such a steady diet. What is more, this surging sea we are immersed in can also stimulate terminal apathy, or cynicism, or feeling overwhelmed, or impotent, and depressed. Have you noticed?

The headlines of today will be old news tomorrow. Yet we are participants in what becomes history on whatever day we choose to sample it. Only it isn't called history. It is called being alive. And it is unfolding in this era at an increasingly rapid rate, to the point of being undigestible and unfathomable.

And although it often seems remote and impersonal and gigantic in scope, we can nevertheless have a small hand in shaping the news by how we "consume" it, by how we hold it and hold ourselves, especially if we choose to respond to it and take an action of some kind, even in the tiniest ways, on the basis of our core human values. Remember (Book 2: *Falling Awake*, Lovingkindness Meditation): when one mind changes, the entire lattice structure of the universe changes in a small way. Small? Yes. Insignificant? Hardly. The seemingly "little" isn't necessarily so little or insignificant. It can be huge. The downstream consequences can be unpredictably consequential. In this era, one person with a smart phone can film an encounter that will be seen and explode on social networks around the world. It is a new way of taking a stand. Of bearing witness. It becomes a political act to participate in this way, to be a node in the network of unfolding events, a news network of one with a potentially vast reach. It is well known from the sciences of chaos and complexity that in any complex, dynamical, non-linear system such as the weather, or the activity of human beings, or the process of thought itself, even the tiniest shift or perturbance can result in changes of enormous magnitude, sometimes occurring at surprisingly great distances from the originating event. Where it concerns the weather, and now even more generally, this principle is known as the "butterfly effect" because it is said that the flap of a butterfly's wings in China can trigger storm systems days later in New England or in other far-flung places. By the same token, as we have seen in the earlier books in this series, tiny but profound shifts in your own body or mind can, over time, lead to major healing. This can happen in the body politic as well. The fate of humanity and everything we hold dear may very well hang in the balance. We see signs of this healing unfolding every day.

But, you might ask, how can we possibly relate to the news mindfully and act responsibly in the face of the enormity of it all and the fire-hose pace at which it comes to us? We are perpetually deluged by information, mis-information, partial information, slanted information, conflicting information, and endless opinions and opining on all sides of all issues, some of it apparently coming from bots, that is, computer programs—not even humans, although programmed by them, one sign of the increasing invasiveness of algorithms and big data in our lives.

Viewed through a slightly different lens, we might say that, whatever news sources we avail ourselves of, we are exposed to what often amounts to a very narrow band of views and perspectives. If we doubt that, all we need to do is take a look at the less-than-mainstream press, or foreign press reports, in the latter case, looking in particular at how other nations perceive us and the events and views we are embroiled in.

Talk about a complex system! How are we to relate to and understand this never-ending stream of different narratives reporting on events unfolding near and far, including "events" that may never have actually happened? And how are we to relate to the fact that, to some degree, this news stream affects us deeply, even if we ignore most of it? It saturates the atmosphere, the landscape and the mindscape. It can exhaust us. It can deaden us. It can gradually erode our dignity, our empathy, and our integrity, whether we know it or not, and whether we like it or not. One way to mindfully guard against this might be to perceive larger patterns that seem to repeat endlessly within the stream, rather than just getting mesmerized by the foam and the spray of the individual details, however absorbing, maddening, or frightening they may be.

We might ask, for instance, what within this endless news stream represents and documents the vibrant health of our nation or the world? What is right with us rather than merely wrong with us? We know that the very fact of its being available to us is huge, compared to societies where freedom of the press is not a constitutionally enshrined and presumably sacred principle, even when it is under widespread and even organized assault. And in parallel, we would also have to ask ourselves: How much of what comes to us as news documents the dis-ease of our nation and world? And how much of it actually masks the underlying dis-ease, and papers over its symptoms?

It is anybody's guess, not that there aren't endless opinions. Obviously, there is no overall "right view," no all-knowing one view, no one way to see, know, or understand it all, just as there is no one way to view and be in relationship to the interior landscape of our own lives, the sensescapes, the mindscape, the bodyscape that we explored directly through our first-hand experiences of these domains in the mindfulness practices described in Book 2, and that, hopefully, you are continuing to cultivate in your own life in a disciplined way, however hard that may be at certain moments. For all of our experiences, inward and outward, are a reflection of the complexity and dynamism of the human enterprise, and ultimately the products of human minds and human hearts in action and all-too-often, sadly, in conflict, including with ourselves.

Within the vast diversity of goings on, at any given time there are always those, as a rule a small minority, who are willing to brazenly and flagrantly bend, break, or attempt to rewrite the laws for their own personal or collective gain. This has never not been a current within politics everywhere. Then there are all those who are maximally disenfranchised, disempowered, who appear to be hopelessly at the mercy of forces they have no direct say in or control over—until, as in South Africa and countless other places, they all of a sudden surprise the world and somehow manage to bring about what seemed impossible the moment before, without resorting to violence.* And there are also those of us, the vast majority, I would say, in this country who perhaps have some sense of empowerment in small ways (which are hugely important all the same) and are just trying to make it through the day and through our lives with a modicum of stability and decency, doing our work and taking care of our families, and trying to know what is happening and what is important to know in this dizzying era of rapid change on all fronts, genuinely caring about the health of the world and feeling its suffering. At the same time, we are feeling, sensing, and knowing that our lives are being deeply affected and challenged by what is going on in the world politically, economically, psychologically, environmentally, and spiritually because we are immersed in it, because we are of it, because it is not separate from us. To "suffer," from the Latin *sufferre*, means to carry, to bear, and we are certainly carrying the world within us and on our shoulders to some degree. And so, we suffer. And at times, it is very hard to bear.

How do we balance our experience of the outer world—when it is mediated not only directly through the senses, but to such a huge degree indirectly through the news and the large political, economic, social, and above all, technological developments that influence and shape our lives—with our interior world, with the inner landscape, so intimately interfaced with the outer as to not really be separate

---

* Although the legacy of Nelson Mandela has fallen far short of the original optimism in the wake of the remarkable peaceful end of apartheid in 1994. One-quarter of South Africans live in extreme poverty and the governing ANC is riddled through with corruption. See https://www.dailymaverick.co.za/opinionista/2018-07-18-mandelas-legacy-can-heal-the-festering-wound-of-the-past/; https://www.nytimes.com/2018/09/30/world/africa/south-africa-anc-killings.html.

from it? Should we minimize our exposure to the outer, even though it affects our lives whether we attend to it or not? Should we pay more attention? Should we pay attention differently? These are the challenges of living in the world nowadays and *not* altogether renouncing the "worldly life," as monastics do in some traditions.

But renouncing it on occasion, taking a break from all the news periodically, can be tremendously refreshing. Some call it a "news fast." Dr. Andrew Weil, a pioneer of Integrative Medicine at the University of Arizona School of Medicine, recommends it to his patients. My experience of it is that, after coming back from a ten-day meditation retreat, or from camping in the wilderness, nothing has changed, even if big events have happened. Years ago, I missed the whole invasion of Afghanistan when I went on a six-week retreat. I could argue that, in one way, I didn't miss a thing. Think in terms of centuries, and you may get my meaning better.

As the world keeps getting smaller and ever more contentious, a line from the eighteenth-century Japanese hermit poet Ryokan keeps resurfacing in my mind: "No news of the affairs of men." How lovely to have no news of the affairs of men for a while. How freeing. Whatever the affairs of state and the news of Ryokan's day, no one knows it now, and few except some historians of Japan in that particular era would even care. But Ryokan, who lived as a hermit, begged for his food in the towns, and played with the village children to the scorn and ridicule of the elders, and made no attempt to do anything memorable that would go down in history, is remembered and revered around the world centuries later for his poetry and wisdom. Here is his poem in full:

*My hut lies in the middle of a dense forest;*
*Every year the green ivy grows longer.*
*No news of the affairs of men,*
*Only the occasional song of a woodcutter.*
*The sun shines and I mend my robe.*
*When the moon comes out, I read Buddhist poems.*

*I have nothing to report my friends.*
*If you want to find the meaning, stop chasing after so many things.*

To stop chasing after so many things…that may be advice worth taking to heart in some way or other. In exactly what fashion would be for each of us to decide for ourselves, depending on who we are and what we most love, and how well we know ourselves.

Recall (see Book 1, Part 1) Rumi's lines from nine hundred years ago:

*The news we hear is full of grief for that future,*
*but the real news inside here*
*is there's no news at all.*

And William Carlos Williams's poignant admonition:

*It is difficult*
*to get the news from poems*
*yet men die miserably every day*
*for lack*
*of what is found there.*

The French have a saying: *"Plus ça change, plus c'est la même chose."* The more things change, the more they remain the same. There is something to it. And yet, when we bring awareness to the present moment, in any moment, that moment is clearly already different by virtue of that very gesture of ours. Simply bearing witness changes everything. It is the power of naming what is, giving voice to what is, and standing in awareness, taking a moral stand, an ethical stand, aligning oneself with one's principles, embodying one's truth, without forcing anything to be different, but without recoiling from the witnessing, even in the face of overwhelming physical force, or social coercion, and perhaps one's own fears as well.

Just bearing witness changes everything. Gandhi knew that. Martin Luther King knew that. Joan of Arc knew that. All three moved mountains with their conviction, and all three paid for it with their lives, which only served to move the mountains even further. They weren't "chasing after so many things." But they did stand for and behind what they knew one hundred percent. And they knew it from the heart at least as much as from their heads. And so have countless others, often nameless, who have shaped and shifted history over the centuries.

You don't necessarily have to surrender your life to bear witness to injustice and suffering and speak truth to power. And just as they were no doubt flawed individuals in some ways, being human, you too don't have to be perfect, whatever that might mean, to take an ethical stance and speak your truth in the face of injustice and the power behind it. Being human will suffice. Of course, integrity and honesty are axiomatic here if we are to be true to ourselves and to the call of the circumstances we find ourselves in in any moment. The more bearing witness while dwelling in openhearted awareness becomes a way of life for more and more of us, the more the world will shift— because the world itself is none other than us. But it is sometimes, more often than not, a long, slow process, the work of generations. And yet, at times, a tipping point is reached that could not be predicted even one moment before. And then things shift, rotate, go orthogonal, and very quickly.

Still, we cannot rely on that happening in the short run. It requires great patience and forbearance to not turn away from the suffering of the world, and yet not be overwhelmed by the enormity of it either, or destroyed by it. It requires great patience and forbearance not to think we can magically fix it all or get it all right just by throwing money at what we see as a problem, perhaps trying to buy influence or allegiance, as is so much the case in politics, or impose our own values on others. Clarity and peace do not come easily to us as individuals, even less so as a society. In one way, we need to work at continually cultivating those qualities of mind and attention that actually *nurture* clarity and peace, selflessness and kindness, even though, seen another way, they are part of us and accessible to us in their fullness even now, and actually, only now. At the same time, we need to recognize our own impulses to perhaps fall into self-righteousness, arrogance, aggression, othering, dominance, or indifference, so as not to be caught by them and, ironically, blindside ourselves.

What is true for the inner world is true in the outer world. Peace, or a change of heart or of view or values, according to the poet-farmer Wendell Berry, is a practice. As he put it, "A change of heart or of values without a practice is only another pointless luxury of a passively consumptive way of life." But it is a practice that we will have to develop for ourselves, as there are no models for how to do it. There is also no single one right way to do it, just as there is no one right way to meditate, or to love. But trusting our own intelligence, and our capacity to read between the lines and not be taken in by appeals to those fundamentalist mind states we can so easily fall prey to, namely only thinking to maximize our own gain or pleasure (we have been calling this "greed"), falling into aversion for what and who we don't like or don't want or respect (we have been calling this "hatred"), and forgetting who and what we are in our deepest nature, and who and what others are, or for that matter, what our country is (we have been calling this "delusion," "ignorance," or "unawareness"), will allow us to make an important difference, a critical difference, however small our own little life and energy field may seem in relationship to the larger forces affecting the world. And as we open our hearts individually through this kind of inner cultivation, through *practice*, we can become examples for each other and inspire each other, thus amplifying our presence and our potentially transformative and healing influence within whatever domains of activity we find ourselves drawn to.

Things change, and it is *not* always *la même chose*, the same old story. Especially if you intend to change the story by waking up and staying awake, and keeping in mind what is most important, and sharing your beauty with others, and recognizing and sharing in theirs, however different it may seem to be from yours, however you choose to pursue it within your comfort zone, and perhaps well beyond your comfort zone too at times. Acts of integrity and goodness inspire such in others. There are any number of fundamentally benevolent acts and humane and important projects occurring in little and big ways everywhere in the world. Each offering, however small, serves as a mirror as well as a beacon, reflecting its own and other kindred offerings of kindness and wisdom and light in all directions.

If we look at human history, we will find that a good heart has been the key in achieving what the world regards as great accomplishments: in the fields of civil rights, social work, political liberation, and religion, for example. A sincere outlook and motivation do not belong exclusively to the sphere of religion; they can be generated by anyone simply by having genuine concern for others, for one's community, for the poor and the needy. In short, they arise from taking a deep interest in and being concerned about the welfare of the larger community, that is, the welfare of others. Actions resulting from this kind of attitude and motivation will go down in history as good, beneficial, and a service to humanity. Today, when we read of such acts from history, although the events are in the past and have become only memories, we still feel happy and comforted because of them. We recall with a deep sense of admiration that this or that person did a great and noble work. We can also see a few examples of such greatness in our own generation.

On the other hand, our history also abounds with stories of individuals perpetrating the most destructive and harmful acts: killing and torturing other people, bringing misery and untold suffering to large numbers of human beings. These incidents can be seen to reflect the darker side of our common human heritage. Such events occur only when there is hatred, anger, jealousy, and unbounded greed. World history is simply the collective record of the effects of the negative and positive thoughts of human beings. This, I think, is quite clear. By reflecting on history, we can see that if we want to have a better and happier future, we must examine our mindset now and reflect on the way of life that this mindset will bring about in the future. The pervasive power of these negative attitudes cannot be overstated.

TENZIN GYATSO, the Fourteenth Dalai Lama
*The Compassionate Life*

# REMINDING MYSELF THAT
## SELF-RIGHTEOUSNESS IS NOT
### HELPFUL

Speaking of negative attitudes, even intending to cultivate equanimity and spaciousness, I notice how easy it is to fall into self-righteousness and indignation as soon as I start thinking about the things I don't like in the world, especially when they seem to stem from either the activity or the inactivity of human beings. I catch myself "personalizing" something that is actually much bigger than individual villains, even though specific persons are playing various, sometimes awful, roles in what is happening at any one moment. What come to mind are the very real injustices, social inequities, and exploitation of huge numbers of people and natural resources, often disguised through the mis-appropriation and corruption of language so that it is hard to discern what is really going on because words themselves have become a kind of surreal newspeak; the boundless harm that comes from waging endless wars to achieve dubious ends by nefarious means; the sense that those in various positions of power and responsibility are often willing to lie outright, dissimilate, fabricate, coerce, manipulate, deny, cover up, buy allegiances, rationalize whatever they are doing, and do whatever they feel necessary to achieve those dubious ends; the increasingly enormous concentration of power and influence and wealth in the hands of a small number of people and of multinational corporate giants who often act as if their interests in power and growth and profits are above all others' and even above the law; to name just a few.

Then I remember: even if all that is true to a degree, and I emphasize, to a degree, usually guessed at but mostly unknown, there are at least two problems with my self-righteous attitude. The self part, and the righteousness part.

I notice that I never feel self-righteous in response to tornados and hurricanes. I never feel self-righteous about the casualties, destruction, and loss caused by flooding, or naturally occurring forest fires, or earthquakes, in spite of the enormous toll they can take in lives and in the mountainous misery of those who survive that usually follows in their wake. Emotions do arise in response to such occurrences, yes, including great sadness, empathy, compassion, and a strong desire to help in some way. But not self-righteousness. Why? I guess because there is no one that I can blame for it, or impute motive to. Earthquakes just happen. So do tsunamis, hurricanes, and other "natural disasters."*

But as soon as there is a "they" behind it, as in "they should have..." or "they shouldn't have..." or "how could they...?" or "why don't they...?"—as soon as there is a sense of agency behind it, along with possible malfeasance, ignorance, greed, irresponsibility, or duplicity, then the impulse to get angry and righteous, impute motive to a "them" and turn them into the problem, even dehumanize them, arises and blossoms forth in me. And it is particularly strong when I feel that "I" am correct, that my views and opinions are grounded in truth, that "I" know what is going on, and can marshal endless corroborating evidence in support of my position. It is even more the case when I "know" that "they" are bending if not breaking the law, dismantling environmental safeguards, trampling on the Constitution, bullying other countries or bribing them, or willfully and systematically concentrating what feels like illegitimate power and influence

---

* But of course, we now know that global warming due to human activity is a direct cause of more frequent and more severe storms, more frequent and severe flooding due to sea level rise, and more frequent and severe forest fires globally.

and wealth and arrogantly exploiting their positions as public servants. And my self-righteousness is an equal-opportunity employer—it can condemn folks on all sides of all issues in all cultures, far and wide, even though I don't know them from Adam, or their cultures and mores.

And there is another problem with my self-righteousness as well. All the things I am objecting to have been going on for centuries. I notice, perusing an outline of early Chinese history in a book of Chuang Tzu's writings, the author of the poem at the end of this chapter, that in approximately 2205 BCE, a man named Yü is described as the "virtuous founder of the Hsia Dynasty," and that, in 1818 BCE, four hundred years later, a man named Chieh, is described as "the degenerate terminator of the dynasty." There have always been cycles of relative tranquility and overriding mayhem, of relative security and rampant insecurity, of relative honesty in public affairs and flagrant dishonesty, of relative goodness and unequivocally evil actions. We can make it personal, blame it on specific individuals, and also take it personally, but it goes much deeper than that. Perhaps we are all players in some dream movie that only ends when we realize that it is we who are keeping the dream going, and that what is most important is for us to wake up. Then all the nightmare characters within the dream may evaporate without having to feed it to keep the dream going and make it work out a certain way.

Do we want to keep cycling in this dream sequence by taking sides in the usual dualistic for-or-against struggle, and fight for the best temporary outcome we might manage to get, even as we stay within the dream and sooner or later, will encounter once again the "degenerate terminator" in the form of a Hitler, a Stalin, a Pol Pot, a Saddam Hussein, a Pinochet or some other horrific personification or faceless spasm of ignorance capable of galvanizing and spreading that virus by appealing to and inflaming fear, hatred, and greed in vulnerable and dissatisfied people? Or do we want to wake up, and thereby dampen and perhaps even extinguish these cycles altogether by inviting in an entirely different, orthogonal understanding of the dream itself, the root of the dis-ease, into our consciousness, and by finding ways to catalyze a healthier dynamic equilibrium that recognizes ways to work with and keep in check those more self-centered, greedy, and aversive impulses in the mind that drive so many of our actions as individuals, and therefore, of so many of our public institutions, and which, sooner or later, always seem to seduce us back to sleep or into trance? Or is it not a matter of either/or but of both together, because they are not actually two distinct features of the world but paradoxically, inter-embedded, one seamless whole?

You see the dilemma. Self-righteousness is not helpful, however understandable it may be, and on whatever side or issue it may fall. It is not helpful because it assumes that things "should" be happening differently. But the truth of it is that they are happening the way they are happening. This is it, right now, and there is only now. Should or shouldn't is irrelevant, part of a story we are telling ourselves that may be blinding us to more imaginative and truer ways to see the situation and to interface with it that might make a real difference, move the bell-shaped curve a bit, catalyze an orthogonal rotation, perhaps name if not put an immediate stop to madness and injustice, as opposed to just changing the cast of characters but keeping the same unexamined, misunderstood, and crazy overall script. The latter is tantamount to rearranging the deck chairs on the *Titanic*, then building another one after it sinks, then rearranging the deck chairs again.

We desperately need to learn to trust our direct experience of things, to conjure up the courage to stand inside our convictions based on wise discernment and clear seeing rather than on ideological grounds or venal political correctness. Maybe we need to teach ourselves and let the world teach us how to rest in a brave openness, perceiving what lies behind the veils of appearance and of misinformation, and also beyond our own blindnesses, wishful thinking, and tendencies to turn everything into black or white, good or bad, and lose touch with the degreeness of things.

Yet, within all of this, we still need to ground ourselves in what we are seeing and sensing. We still need to feel our way into what we might *do*, what we might actually engage in that could make a difference in the world yet without falling into either our small-minded, fear-based self, with all its problems, or into righteousness, which suggests that we are more morally upright than others, somehow purer, more enlightened, without the taint of guilt or sin, that we are the ones who know. The more we say it or think it, the more likely we are to believe it, and then it becomes another reified notion, an impediment to the very freedom and honesty and true morality we are advocating for others and claiming we live by and enjoy ourselves. You can just feel how dangerous that kind of thinking is, especially if we are unaware of it, because that is just what everybody feels, no matter what side of an issue they fall on. "I am right and they are wrong." "I know what is right, and they don't." "What is wrong with them?" Then we start attributing motive.

So are you right when you think you are right? Are they wrong when you say they are wrong? Soen Sa Nim (see Books 1 and 3) used to say, "Open your mouth and you're wrong." And yet, you, we, all of us, have to open our mouths. And sometimes we do have to act, even in the face of complexity and uncertainty, for complexity and uncertainty are part and parcel of the nature of reality itself. What *can* we do? That koan is a worthy meditative practice, and it is a worthy political practice. Can we stay with the not knowing and wake up to something new and daring and imaginative and healing beyond the confines of reactive, unexamined, and highly conditioned thought processes and the grip of afflictive emotions, particularly fear? Can we find ways to embody goodness, a true inner and outer strength, especially in moments of crisis and challenge, and at the same time drop the righteousness, which is both corrosive and corrupting?

Just thinking about things in some ways can trigger self-righteous indignation. Thinking about the same things in other ways opens the way to imagination and creativity, to openheartedness, to mindful and heartful action.

But the self is its own construct, and even if the facts are clear, what we do about a particular situation that triggers self-righteousness in us often is not. "We" can be as ignorant in our indignation as "they" are in their "nefarious machinations," whoever they are, and whoever we are. Don't you already know this in your heart of hearts, someplace deep down? Perhaps something better and wiser is required, more relational, a less dualistic way of seeing, one that does not reify the sense of "us" versus "them," or its kissing cousin, "good" versus "evil," quite so fast, or that sees even that and can hold it gently in awareness, if the impulse in us is so strong that it arises on its own with a lot of emotion in spite of our knowing better. Then maybe, just maybe, we might find ways not to be torn apart by conflict in our own thinking and feeling, and to act wisely and bravely to move things in a direction of healing, of moving from dis-ease and imbalance to greater ease and balance and harmony. In a word, a politics of wisdom and compassion, nurtured through mindfulness and lovingkindness. It would mean a true caring for, protecting, and honoring of the body politic, a commitment to ask the most of it and of ourselves rather than the least, and to trust that clear seeing is the road to true security, and to long-term harmony and balance.

*

*If a man is crossing a river*
*And an empty boat collides with his own skiff,*
*Even though he be a bad-tempered man*
*He will not become very angry.*
*But if he sees a man in the boat,*
*He will shout at him to steer clear.*
*If the shout is not heard, he will shout again,*

*And yet again, and begin cursing.*
*And all because there is somebody in the boat.*
*Yet if the boat were empty,*
*He would not be shouting, and not angry.*

*If you can empty your own boat*
*Crossing the river of the world,*
*No one will oppose you,*
*No one will seek to harm you.*

CHUANG TZU (Third-century BCE)
*Translated by Thomas Merton*

# POLITICS NOT AS USUAL IN THE TWENTY-FIRST CENTURY

*Whoever relies on the Tao in governing men*
*doesn't try to force issues*
*or defeat enemies by force of arms.*
*For every force there is a counterforce.*
*Violence, even well intentioned,*
*always rebounds upon oneself.*

*The Master does his job*
*and then stops.*
*He understands that the universe*
*is forever out of control*
*and that trying to dominate events*
*goes against the current of the Tao.*
*Because he believes in himself,*
*he doesn't try to convince others.*
*Because he is content with himself,*
*he doesn't need others' approval.*
*Because he accepts himself,*
*the whole world accepts him.*

LAO TZU (*Tao Te Ching*) Fifth-century BCE
*Translated by Steven Mitchell*
(*Pronouns in the above as you care to use them.*)

Imagine a politics grounded in mindfulness. Imagine a governing mind set and democratic process that knows and honors that "the universe is forever out of control and that trying to dominate events goes against the current of the Tao," not because this phrase wound up being carved on some government building, but because it had been experienced firsthand through the cultivation of mindfulness by large numbers of people in our society. Our decision-making, even our view of our self-interest, would be radically different if it were held in accord with such an understanding, and with that kind of wise humility. Then consensus and action might come, to a much higher degree than they do now, out of wisdom and compassion and out of an understanding of the gap between appearances and how things actually are, with our actions directed toward the actuality rather than the appearance. Such actions would shape what all communities and constituencies hope for in true governance, hope for from a wise democracy, namely a genuine inquiry into the inner and outer needs of its constituents and of the greater society in which life, liberty, and the pursuit of happiness unfold.

Of course, the genuine needs of a society are always multiple and often in some degree of conflict with each other for limited resources. A more mindfulness-based political process would still no doubt be highly chaotic, contentious, and spirited. But it would also be one in which we might place our trust with greater confidence because we are ultimately trusting in ourselves through one another, and for good reasons that might be far better recognized and honored by all concerned than they are now.

When we use the phrase "politics as usual," it usually means that we are fairly cynical about politics, often times understandably so since it seems based more on mortal warfare between intransigent ideological camps than about serving the greater good. Maybe what we need for this era is really a politics not as usual, marching to a different drummer, or maybe not marching at all, but rather flowing, approached with an intentionally orthogonal mind set, one that keeps in mind the "realities," but, at the same time, keeps in mind as well the primacy of interconnectedness, and the sense of us all being participants in this one body of the world. If we experienced our interconnectedness more intimately through the actual practice and cultivation of mindfulness, we might more readily realize that all our self-centered motivations and impulses are limiting our capacity to perceive the larger picture and how we might be of real use. We would see that small-minded motivations and views are a source of great pain, for both ourselves and others. Greater wisdom and compassion and more effective allocation of resources to catalyze and further benevolent action would spring naturally from such a perspective. Politics itself would become a transformative and healing consciousness discipline. The first people to benefit would be the politicians themselves, from the satisfaction of doing the right thing for the right reasons. But ultimately, the entire world would be the beneficiary.

This may be the unique challenge of our species and of our time: to respond to the possibilities of our own true nature as human beings because we can imagine them, because we can know them, and because we see, perhaps as never before, the potential consequences of *not* responding, of remaining through mere inertia in our consensus trance state, of not waking up, not coming to our senses. The fate of our children and grandchildren, of future generations, and of our species itself may, without exaggeration, very well hang in the balance—not in some far-off future, but perhaps in the next few generations, much sooner than we might imagine.

For, much as we do know goodness and beauty through our own direct experience if we are willing to pay close and gentle attention in our lives, we also know the other side of the matter, that we can all be blinded by our own minds, especially when we mis-perceive the reality of things and are overcome by destructive emotions, especially fear and greed, out of which all the others flow. At such times, we literally and metaphorically contract, and are thereby diminished. The decisions we make in those contracted mind states, the things we say and what we do can wind up creating a good deal of harm, both to ourselves and to others. A lack of intimacy with our own interior landscape of mind and body and therefore a lack of direct familiarity with how it shapes our choices and behaviors, literally from moment to moment, can compound the damage over time, creating ever greater disharmony, disquiet, and dis-ease.

This is still the case even if, maybe especially if, the danger that we collectively perceive ourselves to be in is very real. And it is the case even when the opportunities that we perceive for ourselves and hope to pursue are also real. The interpretation, even the existence and nature of that danger and those opportunities, are still products of our sense perceptions and the activities of our own minds, and so admit a range of ways of being seen and known, depending on the qualities of mind that are being brought to bear on whatever is arising under particular circumstances, especially trying ones. We are all at risk of a reflexive physical, emotional, cognitive, and spiritual contraction in the face of a perceived threat—and that risk is always seriously compounded by our conditioning and the dominant but tacit assumptions of our own culture, especially if as a culture, we in the United States are suffering since 9-11 and its enduring aftermaths, from chronic post-traumatic stress, which we certainly still are.

This is where mindfulness comes in, since, as we have seen, it can be of use on any and every level to refine our capacities for seeing and knowing the actuality of things, underneath their appearances and our own impulses to contract into myopic mind states just when we most need clarity and dispassion. The more mindfulness becomes a heartfelt practice and priority in the world, the more we will wind up increasing the likelihood that we will *respond* to difficult situations in measured, imaginative, and thus, truly powerful ways rather than *react* reflexively in the usual habitually contracted ways. We will be more likely to be proactive in tapping into and releasing new, creative, and more effective and compassionate energies that themselves can catalyze transformational changes in individuals, organizations, and nations that are now primarily and myopically governed by politics as usual.

I am reminded of a description of the martial art of aikido I came across a long time ago but have never forgotten. Paraphrasing: If someone attacks you, he is already out of his mind in a certain way, has already surrendered his own point of independence and balance by the very irrationality of that aggressive act. If you do not succumb to fear and lose your own equanimity and clarity, but rather, enter into and blend with the attacking energy while maintaining your own balance and center, you can use the attacker's intrinsically unbalanced energy and momentum against himself with an economy of effort, doing the least harm and the greatest good. You blend with the opponent, moving him around your own center and thus neutralizing his attack. This can be accomplished with wrist locks and subtle shifts in position almost without you touching him. Yet he is undone, and has no idea how it even came about. Metaphorical aikido may be even more powerful.

Imagine utilizing your power, which you might not think you even have, in such conscious ways in the face of aggression and challenges of all kinds, at all levels in our world, predicated on the recognition that an opponent, an "attacker" or potential "attackers" have already demonstrated a huge weakness and imbalance by the aggressive and therefore irrational or deluded nature of their very act or intention. That is, if we don't lose our own minds as a reaction to others losing theirs, as so often happens, which is how anger begets anger, and violence more senseless violence.

There have always been individuals and groups that have been committed to more humane and benevolent ways of defining and realizing the highest means and the most meaningful ends in various human enterprises, to say nothing of the innate possibilities of being surprised by unpredictable positive outcomes when the process itself, as in true dialogue (see Book 3, Dialogues and Discussions), has integrity and we trust in it without trying to force particular outcomes. *Social entrepreneurship*, such as the development of the vehicle of microcredit, through which progressive banks can make millions of successful small loans to poor people in places like Bangladesh and elsewhere to start small businesses and lift their standard of living, is one notable example of this kind of imaginative "aikido" on the world, in this case, in proactively confronting the forces behind extreme poverty and lack of opportunity and finding ways to "enter" and "blend," to stand at the heretofore unperceived fulcrum of a huge dilemma and let things rotate around the newly introduced element to good effect. Examples abound throughout the world. What is changing now is the growing recognition, already widespread, that the inner and outer landscapes of mind and world interpenetrate, and that we have to come to know and tend, as a gardener tends a garden—at the institutional level as well as in our individual lives—our own motivation and thoughts and emotions and the economic and social factors that influence them in order for even the best of intentions to be effectively realized.

\*

No matter how well informed any of us are or are not on any specific issues, it is a safe bet that, in any given moment, our leaders usually don't have access to the complete story of what is happening either. They are frequently caught having to respond to and juggle unfolding events without fully knowing what is going on or the consequences of particular actions they might take, especially if they are not seeing with eyes of wholeness but are more concerned with safeguarding particular narrowly defined interests, whether economic or geopolitical, or merely their own reputations and above all, with re-election.

In the political arena, as in medicine, decisions often have to be made moment by moment and day to day on the basis of incomplete information and major uncertainty. It comes down to reading patterns within unfolding events and relating them to past experience, to intuition, to weighing the odds, and balancing contingencies and ratios of benefits to risks. These are all judgment calls requiring ongoing awareness, discernment, and integrity. But unfortunately, without awareness and an understanding of what one's true "self-interest" might be—perhaps keeping in mind the interrelationship between self and other and thus nurturing a larger and more "selfless," less self-centered motivation—such decision-making is also inevitably swayed by ideology, political allegiances, and the demands of special interest groups and narrow constituencies one feels beholden to. The impulse to approach things with a more dispassionate and broad-based awareness—coupled with discerning inquiry, a desire for healing, and a commitment to what used to be called, quaintly, *the commonweal*, the well-being and health of our society and world and every individual that inhabits it—can be easily overshadowed, if not completely lost.

Those engaged in the everyday business of politics, even the best of politicians and statesmen/women, and understandably so, are often impelled to put their spin on whatever they think we should be think-ing, rather than being more transparent and honest about their biases and inviting us to make our own decisions. It is so easy to forget that "the universe is forever out of control, and that trying to dominate events goes against the current of the Tao." Unfortunately, their analy-ses of situations are perpetually at risk of being tainted by narrow self-interest and ideology, in addition to the enormity of having to respond to so much complexity and to the uncertainties and high stakes associ-ated with making particular choices, then taking the risk of standing by those principled choices because it is the right thing to do, thereby elevating the conversation, educating their constituencies rather than pandering to them, and being honest, even if it means losing the next election. In the worst cases, of course, the temptation is to slant or obscure or deny the true state of affairs to such a degree that it is tan-tamount to dissimulation or outright lying to the very people they are meant to represent, or appealing to their basest instincts.

In medicine, there is a special word for such an attitude and the behavior and decisions that can flow from it. It is called *iatrogenic*, signifying a condition or problem brought about by the witting or unwitting malfeasance or inaction of the doctor or, more largely, of the health care system itself.

Many prevalent attitudes and practices of politicians would be considered iatrogenic, even criminal, were they taking place in medicine. Unfortunately, in politics, the family of the patient, namely every single one of us, is usually kept in the dark, and only told what those in charge want us to think, often playing on our deepest fears and attributing the source of "salvation" to their own ideas, policies, personality, and party. As ordinary citizens, we may not know much, if anything, of what is actually going on at any particular moment.

On the other hand, as Yogi Berra once famously put it, "You can observe a lot by just watching," and as Bob Dylan famously sang, "You don't need a weatherman to know which way the wind blows." In the same vein, Abraham Lincoln said: "You can fool some of the people all of the time; all of the people some of the time; but you cannot fool all of the people all of the time." Thank goodness for that, although Lincoln said it long before digital algorithms that have the potential to shape our interface with reality without our even knowing it. But that won't stop some candidates for office from trying to fool (or convince) enough people to get elected or re-elected when their motivation is primarily driven by greed or fear or hatred, thereby pandering to the fear of others, thereby undermining rather than uplifting the democratic process. Unbridled capitalism thrives on those all-too-human motivations of greed, fear, hatred, and delusion. Yet even within capitalism, there are incipient movements toward nurturing a more *caring economy* coming to the fore. And why not? It is long overdue.*

If politicians knew, deep down, from firsthand experience, that

---

* See for example, Singer, T. and Ricard, M. (eds.). *Caring Economics: Conversations on Altruism and Compassion Between Scientists, Economists, and the Dalai Lama*, Picador, New York, 2015; Yunus, M. *A World of Three Zeros: The New Economics of Zero Poverty, Zero Unemployment, and Zero Net Carbon Emissions*, Hachette Books/Perseus, New York, 2017.

there is no permanent self-existing "them" to hold on to power, they might just remember or realize that no matter how famous or powerful they become, even if they become president, or become a two-term president, they are only around for a brief moment, their power and their reputation evanescent, the good they can do limited, but the harm they can cause immense.

A healthy awareness of such ironies might motivate our representatives to do the right thing for the right reasons more of the time, and perhaps even to find ways to speak about things that would galvanize their constituents to expand the scope of what they consider their own true self-interest. Perhaps, with the mind more aware of the endemic pull of self-serving considerations and the dangers of losing touch with the core of one's own being, politicians would be able to articulate their positions so well that we would actually understand how they were seeing things and recognize the wisdom in it, or at least, give it a chance, and really support them out of respect, even affection. There have been many instances when such has happened in our past in big and little ways. One example: when President Eisenhower, a huge military hero, having been commander in chief of Allied Forces during World War II, warned the nation of the dangers of a growing military-industrial complex, capable of setting its own agenda and dominating both foreign and domestic policy. It was a remarkably prescient prophecy. Unfortunately, since his time, the military-industrial complex has only mushroomed to behemoth proportions. The international arms business itself is seeding, feeding, and capitalizing (every pun intended) on conflicts large and small throughout the world. It strongly affects our national views and priorities and decisions to this day. Eisenhower would be mind-blown by the pervasive toxicity of its global influence.

I am not advocating some kind of wide-eyed utopian perspective here. I am reminding us of the power of honesty and wholeheartedness, and of trusting in the goodness of all of us radiating through in larger measure when it is actually embodied by those in leadership positions. Leadership positions in government are highly privileged opportunities to contribute to the safety and well-being of the country and those they represent, accorded to specific individuals for a limited time by us, "the people." Such positions are always, at least in principle, accompanied by sacred responsibilities toward the governed. They need to be taken on as such. That is a practice that takes ongoing effort, not mere lip service. It also takes facing the fact that all too often, when the truth is spoken, it is as if it hadn't been. Few seem particularly interested in hearing it at first, so much are we all caught up in, entranced, and mesmerized by our own self-centered preoccupations, when it is the nature of that very self that needs to be brought into question, along with what it would take to bring about true individual and social well-being.

We certainly could benefit from greater wisdom emanating from those in leadership positions. But since to a large extent, they are us, in the sense of being a significant reflection of the zeitgeist and the mindscape of the society, any shift toward waking up and coming to our senses will need to unfold across the entire society and will likely be multigenerational. Thus, we have to be in it for the long haul. On the other hand, we do not know how much time we have, given the toxicity and potentially untoward and devastating consequences of mindlessness and selfing writ large in the world as the twenty-first century approaches its third decade. Still, there are already increasing signs that mindfulness is taking hold and is likely to continue to deepen across the country and globally as more and more people from every walk of life, belief system, and political persuasion adopt this simple way of being in relationship with experience, with life unfolding. This ascendancy of mindfulness, inwardly and outwardly, has the potential to tip us as a nation toward greater sanity and well-being, especially since it is becoming increasingly understood in a more than merely conceptual way that there is only the appearance of a difference between the inner and the outer. From the non-dual perspective of wholeness, they are one, or even better, as Suzuki Roshi once said in another context, "not two, not one."

One possible bright light in this regard: in 2015, the Parliament in the UK issued an all-party Parliamentary report they entitled *A Mindful Nation—UK* which called for a major investment of time and money into mindfulness training and evaluation in four major areas of their society: health, education, business innovation, and criminal justice. This came about because in the preceding three or four years, an MBSR-like course in mindfulness was offered to members of the House of Commons and the House of Lords, and separately, to their staffs. This initiative was the brain-child of several people associated with the Oxford University Center for Mindfulness, in particular, Mark Williams, one of the cofounders of mindfulness-based cognitive therapy (MBCT) and Chris Cullen, an educator and mindfulness teacher. As of 2018, over 200 members of the House of Lords and the House of Commons have taken this very popular program, which now has a wait list to get in. Several hundred staff have taken a parallel program as well. Nothing remotely like this has ever happened in the history of politics, at least in the West in modern times. It is a sign of an emerging confluence of ancient meditative wisdom—meditative practices emphasizing the development of mindfulness and heartfulness/compassion that have been re-languaged, universalized, and shown in many scientific studies within the past several decades to have demonstrable positive effects on the body and mind and society more broadly—with mainstream governmental bodies whose members are trying to find new ways to deal with the challenges and pressures they face personally in their work (including depression and anxiety), while at the same time, looking for and hopefully finding new and more effective ways to govern the country that that might contribute to optimizing its health on a range of fundamental measures of national well-being, far beyond mere GDP.

Sweden and the Netherlands also have longstanding mindfulness programs in their parliaments.

In 2017, the Mindfulness Initiative in the UK Parliament hosted a day-long visit of Parliamentarians from fifteen different countries who were either interested in this experiment and hoping to bring some version of it back to their own countries, or who were already doing it in their parliaments. Mindfulness teachers from many of those countries also attended. As a result of that meeting, mindfulness is now being taught and practiced in the *Assemblé Nationale* in Paris, France, and in a number of other countries.

In the United States, Representative Tim Ryan, at the time of writing an eight-term Democrat from the 17th Congressional District in Ohio and a devoted practitioner of mindfulness and yoga, wrote a book, published in 2014, called *A Mindful Nation: How a Simple Practice Can Help Us Reduce Stress, Improve Performance, and Recapture the American Spirit*. Maybe his presence in the Congress of the United States will ultimately result in a rhizome of practitioners who will work to redefine politics itself so that it tilts more toward benefiting all. Of course, this would have to be done in a nonpartisan, non-dual way—i.e., not Republican or Democrat, red or blue, right or left, merely human. While from one vantage point, this may seem preposterous and grossly utopian, from another vantage point, we may be approaching an inflection point where the preposterous becomes the actuality, as we wake up and come to our senses as a nation and as a planet. Even a little bit would be hugely significant. We have only to begin, which we already have. The practice and the promise of liberation from profound suffering, and the deep confidence in our true nature as benevolent and loving human beings when all is said and done, will do the rest. None of us will be able to "figure this out" merely through thinking. It will require tapping into other dimensions of our intelligence—above all, the open-hearted clarity of wisdom, of awareness itself

# LESSONS FROM MEDICINE

Just as there are few cures in medicine, in spite of all that is known about biology and disease, there are even fewer cures or quick fixes in the domain of the body politic. We work with the world as we find it and as we inhabit it, realizing that our understanding of events and our ability to shape outcomes are always limited, sometimes humblingly so. But, as we have discovered in medicine, that does not mean that profound healing cannot take place if the situation is met in ways that embrace the full spectrum of inner and outer resources for working even a bit more selflessly and orthogonally with what is, with things as they are, especially in the domain of the human mind and heart. The same is possible for the body politic. It too can be approached from a perspective of healing and transformation rather than merely fixing and curing, especially when the fixes can be potentially damaging to the patient and to the very potential for healing.

That is precisely what the movement of mindfulness in various parliaments around the world is trying to accomplish. Obviously, it is what we might call, relatively speaking, a "top down approach." At the same time, a certain mindful political organizing is going on more broadly in communities worldwide, in the United States through groups such as the Me Too movement, Black Lives Matter, and many others. If we are all cells within the one body politic of a country or the larger body of the planet itself, then the health of every one of those cells needs to be optimized. Everybody's health and vital interests need to be met, recognized, and taken into account, while at the same time, we hold the larger interests of the well-being of the whole in mind as well, and protect them to whatever degree is consistent with the allegiance we pledge, as Americans, to the notion of "liberty and justice for all." Just like the meditation practice itself, this is simple but far from easy.

The limits of possible synergies and collaborations between bottom up and top down movements are unknown, but the world is crying out for attempts to heal our society and world through such inclusive mindfulness-based approaches. Even a little mindfulness, because it is so potent and potentially transformative, can go a long way toward dissolving or mitigating many of the barriers to effective resolution of the enmities, disputes, and thorny issues that have dogged and plagued the human enterprise for millennia, including the endemic objectifying and mistreatment of women. Such healing is virtually an imperative in a world that is now so interconnected, so densely populated, so resource-threatened and environmentally stressed, and bleeding so profusely from endless wars and conflicts, terror, genocide, and the huge mass-migrations that have followed directly as a consequence that the very core of its well-being and health is threatened by these chronic diseases. In the past forty years, Americans have learned to participate in appreciating, refining, and sustaining their own health and well-being to a degree that was unthinkable just a generation ago, when you just accepted what the doctor said and never questioned his or her judgment (and there were very few hers in those days). It was unquestioningly assumed that the patient would be a passive recipient of care, and simply needed to follow "doctors' *orders.*" It was not uncommon to conceal a cancer diagnosis from a patient and only tell the family—the thought being that it would only make the person with the diagnosis feel bad unnecessarily. Now we have a Patient's Bill of Rights to safeguard the dignity of the patient from condescension and worse, and to protect the sanctity and confidentiality of the doctor/patient relationship. Not that dignity, sanctity, and confidentiality aren't still compromised all too often, particularly in the incredibly time-pressured and litigious atmosphere in which medicine is now being practiced, and in how much medicine is influenced by drug companies and other special interest groups. Various "market pressures" have compelled doctors to see more and more patients in less and less time, leading to dissatisfaction and malaise all around, on the part of both the patients and the doctors. Medicine itself is suffering and in need of radical healing.

Nevertheless, perhaps even unbeknownst to these larger forces but flowing within them all the same, a significant movement to shift the culture of medicine to a more patient-centered, relationship-centered, and participatory perspective has been taking place. Mind/body medicine in general, and mindfulness-based strategies in particular, under the umbrella paradigm and practices of *integrative medicine,* have been in the vanguard of this cultural shift for over a decade now. Ultimately though, all such qualifiers will need to be dropped. In the end, there is only *good medicine.* And that should be as good as it can be, for everybody.

Is this radical reorientation of medicine damaging the delivery of high quality medical care? Of course not, although in the old days of "the doctor knows best," such a shift in orientation would have been seen as eroding the stature and authority of the physician, and bad for health care. But to the contrary, this change in the culture of medicine and how it is practiced promises to significantly enhance the options and the quality of care for patients and families alike. It is also more satisfying for the doctors, since they now can be—in concert with the other skilled members of the health care team, such as nurses, social workers, physical therapists, psychologists, occupational therapists, nutritionists—more often than not *in partnership* with their patients rather than in a predominantly authoritarian and therefore more isolating relationship.

In fact, in spite of all the problems with medicine and health care nowadays, and those problems are legion, enormous strides have been made toward a more patient-centered and participatory medicine, in which the patient and the physician and the health care team all have their assignments and roles to play, and in which there is, ideally, an informed and honest give-and-take among the parties that changes creatively as things unfold over time. In this model, everyone, including the patient, especially the patient, is working to move the patient toward greater levels of health and well-being and comfort at every age and stage of life to whatever degree possible, right up to the very end of life. Alternative views and approaches to treatment, backed increasingly by credible research, are now a more welcomed part of this process than ever before, and potential synergies between more traditional and more integrative treatment approaches are being recognized and optimized wherever possible, as an increasingly informed public turns to different, often orthogonal perspectives and approaches when faced with health crises that standard medicine heretofore has only dealt with in limited and sometimes grossly unsatisfying ways. Such approaches are now slowly making their way into the standard curriculum as well as into elective offerings in medical schools across the country as a result of the passion and interest of growing numbers of imaginative and caring clinical practitioners in medical centers everywhere. Hospitals themselves are becoming more welcoming environments, more *hospitable*, we might say.

If such profound transformative currents can change the face of medicine in less than one generation, even in a time of crisis in the health care system, driven as they have been to a large degree by "consumer demand," they can also happen, to some degree at least, in politics, also driving by consumer demand, so to speak. Politicians may be highly expert in particular areas, as are physicians and all other professionals, and they may be privy to information we have no access to. Yet they are not omniscient. Their judgment may not be any better or wiser than our own in certain matters. Yet they are vested for a limited time with the authority and responsibility to participate in various ways in critical decision-making to preserve and further the well-being and security of the country and regulate and protect its various homeostatic processes, such as the economy; the rule of equal and impartial treatment under the law—and the need to look at who those laws may protect or favor, and who they don't protect—the education, welfare, and safety of its citizens; diplomatic, trade, scientific, and cultural relationships with other countries; and the natural resources of the environment. But by the very nature of their calling, politicians are perpetually at far higher risk than doctors of becoming caught up in conflicting interests, such as the desire to do good measured against the desire to get re-elected and keep their job and thereby extend the opportunity to serve the greater good; or the constraints of the age-old *quid pro quo* "deals" seemingly necessary to get anything accomplished at all.

If we shift frames for a moment, it is plain to see that such conflicts of interest would severely jeopardize a physician's capacity to make appropriate judgments in regard to their patients. That is why there is a Hippocratic Oath that makes it explicit that the doctor is there to serve the patient's needs above all other pulls and considerations and interests, especially and explicitly personal ones. To embody and protect that selfless relationship with those who are suffering is the core and sacred responsibility of medicine, one that each young doctor vows to uphold.*

Why should we accept anything less where the health of the body politic and, by extension, the health of the world are concerned? Elected and appointed officials take an oath of office as well. Perhaps it is time to pay renewed attention and reverence to those oaths, and perhaps even revise some of them in the light of the pervasive dis-ease that our society and the Earth are experiencing, and in the light of what we are coming to learn about dis-ease and disease, and about our own ability either to compound our problems or heal their intrinsic causes, to whatever degree that may be possible. Maybe those revised oaths should start, as in medicine, with *"primum non nocere…"*: "first do no harm."

---

* That is not to suggest that medicine itself cannot be deeply corrupted. Just think of the travesties of Nazi doctors in the concentration camps in World War II.

Oaths, which are really great vows, if taken to heart as they need to be to be of any import whatsoever, accord us trustworthy reminders and a glide path for staying in alignment and embodying what is most important to living a life of meaning and purpose, often in the face of great obstacles. They call us back to ourselves and remind us of what is, in the end as at the beginning, worthy of our embracing, of our love. No small thing. What would that be for you?

Just as medicine has learned that it has to focus on and understand health as well as disease to appropriately treat a person, so we, as the cells of the body politic, need to act from the side of the health of the society rather than solely reacting to flare-ups or to overt threats of disease. Nor can we perpetually use the constant flare-ups as an excuse for not being able to attend to the true needs of the society and thereby divert our resources away from that attending. At the same time, just as we do in cultivating greater mindfulness in our own lives from moment to moment, in democratically participating in the body politic, it is equally important that we recognize the many energies in ourselves and in others which, out of greed, hatred, fear, or simply ignoring important dimensions of a situation that are therefore not taken into account, pose ongoing dangers to a healthy and harmonious society, whether we are speaking of a family, a community, a country, or the community of all peoples and nations on the planet. In order not to be terminally tainted by these vectors of dis-ease, we need to keep grounding ourselves in ease, in all of the ways we are already healthy, all the while keeping the shadow side of things in both ourselves and others in full awareness. We could call that practicing preventive medicine in politics.

But how do we do that, you might ask? How do we get there?

Simple. There is no "there" to get to. The ease is already here, underneath the dis-ease! The balance is already *here*, inside the imbalances! The light is already here, behind the shadow! We need to remember this, and realize it in the sense of making it real, through the ongoing cultivation of mindfulness, in other words, through practice, which is tantamount to keeping in mind what is most important. The dis-ease itself is only an appearance, albeit, recalling Einstein's phrase, a persistent one, with serious and very real consequences. We all feel it, in some moments and in some years more than we do in others. And some of course, feel its harmful side far more than others, usually as a function of poverty, race, and gender pure and simple. But even these very real elements are not the whole story. For we don't need to *find* our goodness to restore balance, we only need to *remember it*—to reconnect with it, and embody it in our actions.

Simple? Yes. Easy? No.

Ultimately and profoundly, it is *ease* that is the substrate, the ground of our being, as individuals, as a culture, and as a world. We do not always know this, but we can recover it, dis-cover it, precisely because it is already here. It lies at the root of our nature, this dance between dis-ease and ease, between illness and health, whether we are talking about our own body, the body of America, or the world as one body, one seamless whole, one organism really. And for us as a species, nothing is more urgent or more important than that we do dis-cover it. Everything hangs in the balance. Fortunately this ease, this wholeness of being, as we have also been seeing, is right under our noses. It always has been.

If the basic fact is one of dis-ease masking innate ease of well-being, then we need to arrive at a consensus diagnosis of the ailment, however complex it may appear to be on the surface, and however many different opinions there are regarding it, and then explore appropriate "treatments." If we miss the diagnosis, all our efforts to address and alleviate the fundamental underlying dis-ease and the suffering that stems from it will be for naught. We will also be much more susceptible to demagoguery out of our fear and feelings of insecurity and dissatisfaction, stoked, funded, and exploited by groups and perspectives with primarily self-serving agendas and toxic ideologies, but also, if we are honest, evoking or exploiting very real grievances on the part of alienated individuals of all stripes who feel their well-being and their concerns and suffering are not being recognized or addressed, or perhaps are even being betrayed.

It is not that a great deal of what is going on in the world wouldn't benefit from reform, and in some cases radical reform. The world has clearly benefited enormously over the centuries from the efforts of valiant reformers. It is just that we also require something bigger and more fundamental at this point, because a fixing orientation by itself ignores the rotation in consciousness that is necessary for healing the underlying disease and dis-ease. Without it, we are likely to catapult ourselves reflexively into a rescuing, fixing mode, without looking deeply into and understanding more clearly the root causes of our problems, our suffering, our dukkha, and therefore overlooking the need to work with those causal factors up close and personal, in the landscape of our own minds and hearts.

What is more, since what may appear broken to some may not be of any concern to others, the very mind set with which we see and know requires examination, cultivation, and, above all, ongoing conversation and genuine dialogue rather than the noise and haranguing that tend to dominate public discourse. Mindful dialogue (see Book 3, "Dialogues and Discussions") invites true listening, and true listening expands our ways of knowing and understanding. Ultimately, it elevates discourse, and makes it more likely that we will gradually learn to listen to and grow from understanding one another's perspectives rather than just fortifying our own positions and attachments and stereotyping all those who disagree with us. As we grow into ourselves through paying closer attention to our own minds and the minds of others who see things differently, our sense of who we are as an individual expands, and what most needs attention and healing changes for us. We may feel less threatened personally as our view of who we are gets larger, and we see how deeply our interests and well-being are embedded within the interests and well-being of others, and of the whole.

As we have seen (Book 3), when people are considering enrolling in the MBSR Clinic, we often say something along the lines that, from our point of view, "As long as you are breathing there is more right with you than wrong with you, no matter what is 'wrong' with you." We extend this message to people with long-standing chronic pain conditions, heart disease, cancers of all kinds, spinal cord injury and stroke, HIV/AIDS, and to many with less terrifying medical problems but, nevertheless, like these others, with rampant stress and distress in their lives. And we mean it. And, even though they don't and can't possibly know what they are getting into at first, no matter what we tell them, as they cultivate mindfulness formally and informally, they discover that it is indeed the case. As long as they are breathing, there *is* more right with them than wrong with them, no matter what they are suffering from. As they recognize this, and commit to taking the program as a complement to whatever medical treatments they may be receiving, not as a substitute for medical treatment, a large majority grow and change and heal, often in ways they themselves would not have believed possible a short time earlier. The message itself becomes an invitation into the orthogonal, into new ways of seeing and being with things as they are. And it is *the practice* that provides the vehicle and framework for the actual realization of what the invitation is merely pointing to. This growth and change and healing in people with chronic medical conditions has been described and confirmed over and over again in scientific studies over the past forty years.

The same principle applies to the world. No matter what is wrong with it, as long as it is "breathing," there is more right with it than wrong with it. There is a great deal right with it, and with the various "metabolic" functions and homeostatic processes that keep it healthy. Some of this we certainly realize and even appreciate and celebrate from time to time. But much of the health of the world and its peoples is totally ignored, completely taken for granted, or discounted, even abused.

But what does "breathing" correspond to in the body politic? How will we know when the world is close to not breathing and therefore it is already past time to act? Will it be when we can no longer go outside in our cities and breathe the air? Or when our bodies and our children's and our grandchildren's bodies are all carrying an overwhelming burden of toxic chemicals courtesy of the air we breathe, the water we drink, and the food we eat, internal assaults against which the body has no defenses? Or will it be when the global temperatures warm to the point of melting the ice caps and all the glaciers, and flooding our coastlines worldwide, a threat that was so much less apparent when this sentence was originally written fifteen years ago than it is now, in 2018? Or when the periodic genocides on the planet get even larger and more frequent and perhaps closer to home? Or when infectious diseases spread around the world at greater than the speed of SARS or AIDS or Ebola and are no longer containable? Or when terrorism is a regular occurrence in our country? Or will it only be when the things that happen in the movies, such as a nuclear attack on one of our cities, happen for real? Or when AI eliminates millions of jobs? What will it take to wake us up, and for us to take a different, more imaginative, and wiser path?

To face the autoimmune disease we are suffering from as a species, and that we are equally the cause of, we will need, sooner or later, to realize the unique necessity for the cultivation of mindful awareness, with its capacity for clarifying what is most important and most human about us, and for removing the thick veil of unawareness from our senses and our thought processes; its capacity for re-establishing balance to whatever degree might be possible—always unknown; and its capacity for healing, right within this very moment as well as over time. If we have to come to it sooner or later, why not sooner? Why not right now? What is to prevent us from undergoing a planetary rotation in consciousness at this point in time, or at least taking the first steps available to us right now? We could start by paying attention to and honoring what is right with ourselves and the world and pour energy into that, and move on all levels and on all fronts, boldly, wisely, incrementally, toward creating the conditions whereby the complex, self-regulating capacities we have as a society and as a world can settle into a dynamic balance, a balance that our own minds have managed to disturb and disrupt and threaten through unawareness, through avoiding a deep inquiring into what is most important, and thus, ultimately through ignorance.

Even though as a nation and as a planet we are under a great deal of stress, and are suffering massively from dis-ease and diseases, at present these conditions can be worked with, managed, and ultimately will resolve, just as such conditions can resolve or be greatly improved in individuals suffering from chronic medical problems when they are seen and met over and over again with awareness. We might do well to put our energy into that seeing and that knowing, and learn how to inhabit and act out of our ease, to inhabit our true wholeness, which is the root meaning of the words "health," "healing," and "holy." Otherwise, we will not be attending wisely to the dis-ease. If we are not careful, especially where the body politic is concerned, we might wind up fueling its root causes, all the while fooling ourselves into thinking that we are eradicating them.

So clarity in diagnosing what is wrong and what is right with us based on the preponderance of the evidence, even in the face of some uncertainty, which is the case in medicine much of the time, is extremely important. And it is ultimately the responsibility of all of us to do that, not just a few experts. A mis-diagnosis is a mis-perception. And a mis-perception in this domain can have severe untoward, you might even say lethal, consequences.

Here is an instance in which, individually and collectively, we desperately need to perceive what is actually going on in its fullness and investigate where the roots of the pain and suffering actually lie. As in a medical diagnosis, many different approaches can be brought to bear on understanding the root nature and cause of the disease. Then, as with medical treatments, different approaches can be employed as appropriate, on the basis of the diagnosis and the understanding of how that particular pathology unfolds. Some treatment approaches can be deployed simultaneously, some delivered sequentially, in all cases monitored and modulated according to how the patient responds.

In the case of the world, we will need to bring the full armamentarium of human wisdom and creativity to bear on making the correct diagnosis and then on an appropriate and flexible treatment plan to bring about the restoration of health and balance, rather than losing ourselves in desperate but misguided and superficial and mechanical attempts at fixing specific aspects of the underlying disease when we don't actually understand what it is or know its origins, and when we forget that healing is fundamentally different from curing and fixing, and often a more appropriate and a more attainable option. Healing is not a mechanical process that can be mandated or forced. We drift way off course if we are only treating the symptoms of the dis-ease, and reacting to them out of fear rather than out of respect for the patient, the body of the world, the world seen and known as one body, which I suspect we are on the verge of realizing it is. And while individual bodies inevitably do die, life itself goes on. Regarding the planet, it is life itself, both present and future generations, and the health of the natural resources, processes, and mechanisms that sustain it that we are concerned with here.

There is much to be learned from the new medicine that is emerging in this era, a medicine that honors the patient as a whole person, much larger than any pathological process, whether an infection or a chronic disease, disorder, or illness not amenable to cure. It recognizes that each of us, no matter what our age, our story, and our starting point, has vast, uncharted, and untapped inner resources for learning, growing, healing, and indeed, for transformation across the life span; that is, if we are willing and able to do a certain kind of work on ourselves, an inner work, a work of profound seeing, a deep cultivation of intimacy with those subterranean resources we may not remember we have or may not have faith in. In the three earlier volumes in this series, we have seen how drinking deeply from this well can contribute profoundly toward the healing of one's mind, body, heart, and sense of deep connectedness with the world, and toward making a very real, perhaps even comfortable peace with those things in one's life that are not amenable to fixing or curing.

None of this means that mindfulness is some kind of magical elixir or cure. Nor does it mean that mindfulness is the answer to all life's problems, medically or politically. But cultivating intimacy with how things actually are is the first step on the path of healing, whether we are talking about a person or a nation, or all nations and all beings. This kind of wise attention provides a practical, non-naïve way to reclaim our humanity, to be what we already are but have perhaps lost touch with, in a word, to be human, fully human. After all, we do go by the appellation human beings, not human doings. Maybe that itself is trying to tell us something. Maybe we need to inquire into what *being* actually entails. That inquiry might lead us to what being fully human might require of us and what it might offer to us that we have not yet tasted, touched, or developed.

Whether we adopt an autoimmune model, a cancer model, or an infectious model to describe the origin of our collective dis-ease and suffering—and in fact, these approaches are all interrelated, in that autoimmune diseases and their treatments can frequently make the body more susceptible to cancers and to opportunistic infections—it is clear that what seem at first, to the privileged at least, to be tolerable, if not minor and ignorable symptoms of societal disease and dis-ease, such as poverty, denigration, injustice, racism, tyranny, and fundamentalism sooner or later can wind up in the heart of the organism if not attended to in appropriate ways, which includes addressing the underlying dis-ease processes that give rise to and feed them rather than merely masking or temporarily assuaging the symptoms. Of course, that would also include keeping in mind that, as in medicine and health care, prevention is the best policy in governing and in diplomacy.

# THE TAMING POWER OF THE SMALL

We are wont to vilify particularly egregious emergences of ignorance as evil. This allows us to assert categorically our own identification with goodness in contradistinction. It is a gross and ultimately unhelpful gloss, even if there are elements of truth in it. Both views, of others as evil and of ourselves as good, may be better characterized as ignorant. For both ignore the fundamental disease, the one that manifests in human beings when we fall prey to unawareness of the preciousness of life, and wantonly or witlessly harm others in seeking pleasure and power for ourselves. In the Old Testament, in Book of Psalms, evil is often referred to as "wickedness." But perhaps a better rendering would be "heedlessness,"* an inattention to the full spectrum of the inner and outer landscape of our experience. This inattention allows us to artificially separate self from other, the "I" from the "Thou" in Martin Buber's terminology, to de-sacralize the world and thus make it predicated on division, on artificial separation and boundaries, on mere mechanism. In doing so, we forget or never recognize a deeper underlying unity and integration that allows for greater possibility, for the emergence of new degrees of freedom and greater latitude in our maneuverability and conduct, both in our interior lives and within the vast diversity that is the world.

---

* See Fischer, N. *Opening to You: Zen-Inspired Translations of the Psalms*, Penguin, New York, 2002.

This unawareness of interconnectedness is not evil, although the consequences stemming from it can be monstrous, and must be recognized and contained wherever and whenever they arise. This is ignorance, a profound discordance, a fundamental out-of-touchness with basic elements of relationality inherent in being alive, in being human. But such ignorance or unawareness, whatever we choose to call it, can assume the face of evil, and can also cause us to project evil onto others when, in fact, they too are suffering from the same disease of ignoring, disregarding, corrupting, and trampling on what is most fundamental, having perhaps never tasted recognition, benevolence, and connectedness in their own lives, or overriding their experience of them in the service of a narrowly construed self and its desires. We need to name it wherever it can be detected in its earliest stages and act decisively to sequester and deactivate it, much like a virus that can easily infect a vulnerable population.

Yet, there have been numerous instances in our own history in which we have aided and abetted those we later declared to be evil. How many times as a nation have we turned the other way when despots were serving our political or economic interests, or when rampant carnage was being loosed on innocents in unfathomable numbers in lands we had no geopolitical interest in? How many brutal, murderous dictators have we tolerated or supported and supplied weapons to when our leaders felt it was in our national interest to build "strategic alliances"? The list is depressingly long, and in retrospect, hugely sobering. All of that may have been clever realpolitik in the past, or the best we could manage under world circumstances we were powerless to control or not-so-secretly favored. But now, with the world community so entwined and interrelated, such compromises and accommodations of convenience with ignorance, or with evil, if you wish to call it that, can no longer be so easily rationalized and will not be so easily forgiven or forgotten.

As a country, we need to take little steps, maybe even tiny steps, but brave steps nonetheless, in the direction of greater wholeness and greater embodiment of mindfulness and heartfulness if we hope to heal the suffering of the world while contributing less to compounding it. We will need to recognize earlier the roots of that suffering, namely greed, hatred, and ignorance, and act more resolutely to stem the potential harm that always ensues from the delusional grasping for power at the expense of wisdom, kindness and interconnectedness, whether within ourselves or within others. It is important that we not underestimate the power of the tiniest shifts in consciousness at a national level toward greater awareness and greater selflessness. As we have already made note of, the little is not so little. Two women cornering a senator in an elevator on national television, speaking their truth to him at a critical moment and demanding he see them as humans and make eye contact with them can sometimes make a difference. You never know. And you may never know how far the ripples go out, even if your proximal goal is not achieved.

Ancient Chinese culture called it *the taming power of the small*. Gandhi knew that the smallest move or gesture, well thought out and morally grounded, packed huge potential, like the inconceivable amounts of energy contained in the tiniest atom. Martin Luther King, along with many other leaders within the Civil Rights Movement, men and women, some well-known and many broadly unknown, embodied this knowing and mobilized tremendous power out of no power, out of moral persuasion, out of a long-downtrodden people's pride in themselves and the sheer beauty and uplifting, inspiring quality of King's oratory. And of course, the eight-hour workday, child labor laws, gender equality, and desegregation were all won through popular grassroots movements that started small, and that doggedly badgered and perturbed the system, often at huge sacrifice of many anonymous individuals, until it responded and shifted. Those achievements did not originate in the White House or in Congress, which invariably only respond once they are pushed, and pushed hard. Some call it people power. Whatever we call it, its potential for transformation is immense.

The world is always changing. Nothing remains the same. When we align ourselves and our original mind and its innate goodness with the natural unfolding of change itself and the pregnancy of each moment with infinite possibility, gradually, little by little, the world responds. The dynamic, ever-changing lattice structure, or better, the fluxing web of interconnectedness, shifts slightly because of your realignment, your inward shift, your orthogonal rotation in consciousness, and the outward manifestations that stem from it. And you are not alone, even when you think you are. Whether we are so-called ordinary citizens or so-called representatives of the people, mindfulness practice can mean allowing ourselves tiny little tastes of our own presence and purpose, availability and goodness, tiny little tastes of our own wakefulness right here, right now. It can mean sampling such moments many times over, if we can remember to drop in on this moment, however it is, wherever we find ourselves, and so come to know the taste of inward clarity and peace, even as we embrace and aim to extinguish the causes of disregard, of exclusion, of inner and outer harm, of conflict. We can build on such experiences by remembering that it is always an option to stay in touch with and inhabit the present moment *as it is*, and by not losing our minds, easy as that is to do in the face of the challenges and opportunities we face, so often exasperating, so often toxic, so often mindless.

The life of the body politic is at least as complex as the life of the body, yet the former has not had the benefit of millions of years of sculpting and refining through evolution, and the sloughing off of solutions that didn't quite work. If the human species is in its infancy, governance and democracy are even more so. When asked what he thought of Western civilization, Gandhi replied: "I think it would be a good idea." As a species, we are a cosmic experiment in process. The universe could care less how it works out. But we might, if we care about anything larger than our own small-minded gain and transient comfort. And clearly, we do. That is the beauty of our species. We are not to be underestimated. But the only intelligence on the planet that could ever underestimate us is, irony of ironies, ourselves.

# MINDFULNESS AND DEMOCRACY

Improbable as it may sound, the fact that more and more people are meditating these days or find themselves thinking about it and wanting to meditate could be thought of as one indicator of our ongoing collective evolution and nascent development as a democratic society.

The United States of America is a nation that, however imperfectly, rather early on declared its independence from oppression and autocracy—economic, political, and religious—a nation that articulated principles of individual autonomy and basic human rights "for all," that spoke up early for life, liberty, and the pursuit of happiness. Thus it set the stage for an inevitable and continual, if punctuated and grossly ironic evolution in individual and collective consciousness, given its own roots in genocide and slavery. Clearly the consciousness of the native peoples and enslaved Africans knew a very different reality from that of the lofty principles of the white power establishment enshrined in the Declaration of Independence and the Constitution.

For what is liberty, what is freedom, if not the possibility, the right, and even the responsibility of each of us without exception finding our own way, and "way" with a capital W even, in the world— trusting our instincts and experiences, learning as we go, growing as we learn, even from what is most painful and from our own mis-takes and mistakes?

And what is growth metaphorically if not an expanded awareness of oneself in relationship to the larger world and one's place in it, a deeper understanding of the interconnectedness of things and their underlying harmony, even in the midst of chaos, and a deepening ability to live free of those forces, both inner and outer, that cloud our understanding of what is real and fundamental and most important? What is growth metaphorically if not an expanded empathy for others and for the world, a reaching out to suffering by one who already knows suffering intimately, or who could, and knows it? There is a requirement for humility here. Without hard-earned or naturally come-by humility, there can be little enduring wisdom or sustaining of compassion, nor their enshrining in basic laws as a bulwark against gross injustice and tyranny. Whether inward or outward, growth that does not come into harmony with the greater whole is a cancer, a disavowal of wholeness and balance and a major threat to them. Such growth is neither sustaining nor sustainable in a healthy body politic, in a true democracy.

If we allow ourselves to follow a path of evolving consciousness as individuals, in response perhaps to some deep and inchoate yearning for peace and happiness and for a greater freedom from the afflictions of disconnection and distress and dis-ease, sooner or later it will have a profound impact on our relationships with each other and on the society and world we inhabit. It has to.

Peace and happiness are not mere election slogans, commodities to be acquired or conferred. They are qualities that can only be embodied and lived. And they can only be embodied and lived in practice, not merely in the enunciation of principles, however lofty. Thus, here at home, we have seen all those who were originally excluded by law and social mores from participating in and benefiting from the *declaration* of inalienable rights of freedom and self-governance "for all," by fits and starts and through tenacious and courageous struggle transform, in tandem, however slowly and painfully, both our consciousness and our laws—regarding slavery, race, indigenous peoples, women, children, sexual orientation, marriage, even gender identity—as well as our understanding of the enormous suffering of real people and real families occasioned by exploitive institutions and the laws and social conventions that upheld them and still uphold them—that is, until they change and are then, in their new form, hopefully actively and vigorously enforced. We have a long way still to go in this regard.

In an evolving democracy, the list of current social injustices and grievances at any given moment is likely to be a long and endlessly heart-breaking one. Yet the growing goes on too, although often excruciatingly slowly and with huge costs to those who are excluded from the bounty, actively oppressed by the inequities of the status quo, and expected to live for generations off the ironies of rhetoric and the indignities and harm of systematic exclusion and exploitation. It is also at huge cost to those who do the excluding, although they might not recognize it at the time, and to the society that suffers from missing the richness of those streams of human life.

And why should the growing into real freedom not continue and even accelerate, starting right now, if we are true to our principles, however slow we have been until now growing into them as a nation? Everything else is accelerating in our era, especially how fast we go to war. Why not accelerate how fast we go to peace? Just how willing are we to wage peace and actually embody peace and liberty and justice for all? Right now. Why can't we mobilize our collective resources and our collective will to affect that kind of transformation, the kind we claim we believe in and stand for in the world? Why not have a Department of Peace, for instance, as well as a Department of Defense? And why not promote inner peace, tranquility, and wisdom as well as outer peace in the world at the same time? After all, they are not separate. Recall once again Suzuki Roshi's "Not two, not one."

In a society founded on democratic principles and a love of freedom, sooner or later meditative practices of all kinds, what are sometimes called *consciousness disciplines*, are bound to come to the fore, as is happening now as the climate for ever-deepening personal and collective independence, interdependence, and well-being is nourished and blossoms. Democracy by its very nature encourages and nurtures pluralism and a diversity of views. It encourages us to take full advantage of our freedoms, both inwardly as well as outwardly, in the pursuit of happiness. It also encourages us to make our voices heard. In such a climate, we are naturally drawn to inquire into and come to understand ourselves in deeper and deeper ways as individuals, as a society, and as a species. It is part of the ongoing evolutionary process on this planet, however modulated and shaped it has become by our scientific and technological abilities to transform the environment and shield ourselves from certain kinds of risks. It is astonishing, but also heartening and understandable, that Americans in such large numbers have taken to fine-tuning their own minds and thus their lives through the practice of meditation, and that there is such a profound hunger for realizing our wholeness and our freedom, and to not be constrained by our circumstances, whether privileged in one way or another, or far from privileged. This growing interest in meditation practice and its integration into life in all ways is now flourishing in countries throughout the world, even those that are not democracies. It is a rising tide, hopefully one that will continue for decades and centuries. In a small but not insignificant way, whether it will continue or not depends on your commitment and mine to practice mindfulness and embody it in our lives, each one of us. I see it as both a privilege and a profound responsibility.

Of course, democracy can take root and grow in a particular culture only if and when the conditions are ripe. It cannot be imposed from without, any more than we could impose meditation on anybody, even though it too may be intrinsically beneficial under the right circumstances. As a country, we may be committed to nurturing conditions for universal freedom and liberation from oppression, exploitation, and ignorance as best we can for a complex set of reasons and motives that sometimes generate policies that seem to support the exact opposite. But to the extent that we care about true democracy emerging elsewhere, we also have to be patient, waiting for the unseen metamorphosis and inward transformation to take place, nourishing it as best we can, to the degree that we can, yet without forcing the chrysalis to open before its time, at least if we hope for a butterfly to emerge. And not all butterflies look alike.

Since the potential for wisdom, kindness, compassion, empathy, devotion, joy, and love are already folded into our deepest truest nature as human beings, wherever we live on this globe, the conscious development and deployment of these capacities may make the difference between peace and perpetual war, between true security and perpetual insecurity, between rampant dis-ease and true liberation of human society from its own self-destructive tendencies. What do we have to lose by moving more intentionally in this direction, other than those ingrained habits of inattention and perpetual self-distraction that distance us from ourselves and keep us living in perpetual fear, forgetting that we are already whole, already complete, and that our true security is in a healthy body politic, in which we all play a critical role?

It is highly diagnostic of our dis-ease as a country that the *New York Times* feels under such assault that it periodically devotes full-page ads* to saying:

> The truth affects us all.
>> The truth helps us understand
>> The truth can't be ignored.

And then, on the following full page:

> The truth
>> demands
>> our attention.

These are wake up calls. Desperate ones. Is anybody listening? Time to wake up and embody what we most value.

---

* Sunday, July 22, 2018, pp. 9 and 11.

# Talking Vietnam Meditation Blues—A Snapshot from the Past, or Is It the Present? *And* the Future?

I started meditating in the mid-1960s. For someone who grew up on the streets of New York, in Washington Heights, it felt like quite an unusual thing to be getting into. Almost no one I knew meditated. There were very few good books about meditation in English (and those you had to search for in weird "underground bookstores"), and virtually nothing about it in the media. I never thought of meditation as a "counter-culturish" thing to do, in part because the term hadn't quite been invented yet. I guess it felt a bit oriental in a romantic way, a sense that something had been discovered and nurtured for centuries in the "Mysterious East" that was potentially relevant for living fully and well and therefore, might be worth experimenting with.

Earlier brushes with Buddhist and yogic meditation within our culture, among the beat poets in the fifties, some of whom, like Gary Snyder, went to Japan to practice, coupled with the visits to this country of a few luminaries even before that, at the turn of the twentieth century, on the occasion of the first World Congress on Religion that took place in Chicago, planted tiny dharma seeds in this country that sprouted in the sixties. Alan Watts's book *Psychotherapy East and West* was an important catalyst in that nascent experimentation.

I was of the generation that came of age in the mid-sixties, the one that, whether we were students or not, whether we were politically engaged or not, whether we were born to privilege in one way or another, or not, seemed to be experimenting in unusually large numbers with different ways of breaking free from the social conformity that dominated the fifties. We were sometime-confused, sometime-intrepid young explorers on the growing edges of society, America's children really, looking for a kind of clarity, a goodness, a promise we were not finding in the conventional pursuits of success, power, status, fame, and fortune within the capitalist/ corporate/political mainstream dream—especially against the what-could-only-be-described-as-surreal backdrop of the Cold War, and, within that, of the "superpower" that we were waging relentless war day after day and year after year against a small agrarian society with no air force or navy, eventually dropping more bomb tonnage on Vietnam than on all of Europe in World War II. Some of us were looking for a place to stand and to be and to work that had the integrity of a greater awareness of the whole of things, for all the contradictions and paradoxes that we knew or quickly learned are part and parcel of living in this world. We were also incredibly angry and disillusioned about what was going on.

In the meetings of the Science Action Coordinating Committee (SACC) at MIT, which a small group of us graduate students founded in 1968 to bring the issues of MIT's deep engagement in the war and war-related research and weapons development into open conversation and dialogue (see Book 3, *The Healing Power of Mindfulness*, p. 45), we often practiced yoga together on someone's living room floor, then engaged in some sitting meditation as well before we entered into the agenda. It was just a dabbling, but a heartfelt one, a nod to our growing sense that the changes we were trying to catalyze in ourselves and the world weren't just a shift in priorities, or putting a stop to certain kinds of things from going on in our name, but rather a shift in awareness, a rotation in consciousness that felt big to us, even though, compared to the issues and social forces we were facing up to, it also seemed small and improbable.

MIT had two highly celebrated laboratories devoted almost entirely to war-related research, dating back to the Second World War. They had made important contributions to winning that war, including sharing in the development of radar, and the invention of inertial guidance systems to direct gunfire and rockets, as well as to help planes and boats navigate solely by instruments. Part of our student agenda was to engage the MIT community in an extended dialogue around issues that were never spoken of in an open forum in those days, and as part of that, to hold a work-stoppage on campus for one day, in which we were asking people to voluntarily suspend all business as usual, including all teaching, research, and office work, and devote the entire day to dialogue and inquiry within the community about our engagement as an institution in war-related research and the design and development of weapons of mass destruction.

Being MIT students, and thus trained in research and its importance, we had done extensive research on our own to uncover what was actually going on at MIT, information that very few people in the community even knew about. The day-long work-stoppage was meant to be a time for institutional dialogue and inquiry, for listening to one another articulate our various differing views on the relationship between science and technology and their uses and possible abuses in society, including whether a university should be engaged in research and development of such weapons. This was hugely controversial, in part because the country was so polarized around the Cold War and Vietnam, in part because we polarized things even more by calling our work-stoppage a strike. There was a great deal of hullabaloo and inflammatory feeling expressed on all sides in the months leading up to it. But we did pull it off. MIT shut down for a day, on March 4, 1969, to carry on a dialogue on the issue of war-related research.

Parenthetically, several of us who founded SACC encouraged and cajoled some prominent senior members of the MIT faculty to form their own group in support of that day of dialogue and inquiry. The faculty group, in the beginning consisting for the most part of scientists in theoretical physics and biology, needed a lot of help and encouragement in the early stages, or so we thought in our youthful exuberance and hubris. So we helped them to get organized. We even proposed the name that they adopted for their new organization, the Union of Concerned Scientists. The Union of Concerned Scientists (UCS) is still very much in existence today, almost fifty years later. It is a highly respected international organization whose members are some of the most prominent scientists in the world, working on some of the most pressing problems of the world at the interface between science and technology and matters related to food, energy, the environment, security, global warming, and public policy. For us students, it was one more example of never knowing how things are going to unfold but not letting that be an impediment to taking a stand for what we believed in, for its own sake. March 4, 1969, was one of those seminal branch-point moments.

Has the UCS changed the world? Who knows? Is the world somehow better for its being there and not only caring but taking care of some important and scary issues that would not otherwise be getting even the little attention they are getting because of their efforts? I think so. Every little bit counts, often in ways we cannot completely know, especially at the time.

Hoping to convince him to give the opening keynote speech on March 4, 1969, a few SACC representatives went over to the Bio Labs at Harvard to pay a visit to George Wald, who I had known from childhood. The avuncular biology professor was famous for his brilliant and eloquent undergraduate lectures. He had also won the Nobel Prize a few years earlier for his elucidation of the chemical processes underlying vision. George readily accepted our invitation, and proceeded to draft a speech he called "A Generation in Search of a Future." When the day came, he spoke movingly of why he felt that the undergraduates in his hugely popular Nat. Sci. 5 classes at Harvard were becoming more and more disaffected. He covered the most salient elements of the current day, the Vietnam War, the Cold War, the draft, war crimes committed by the United States as well as by our adversaries, and framed them in such a way that the conventional view of them, the need to "be practical" and accept the status quo—the arms race, the endless killing, always rationalized by the aggression of the other side, the sanitized language that speaks evenhandedly and rationally about nuclear war and its consequences—was brought into focus that day and called out as bankrupt, immoral, and absurd. Through his seemingly extemporaneous musings, backed by facts and figures and his own potent moral persuasiveness, he managed to craft an entirely orthogonal view for that era. It felt like a courageous speaking of truth to power, and coming from him and from MIT "on strike," we knew the White House, the Congress, and especially the Pentagon were going to take note of it. It was a talk that moved the audience deeply because, beyond whatever views the individuals listening may have held, they knew that they were hearing what may very well have been a greater truth, articulated and embodied in George's emotionally nuanced and captivating way. George spoke a good deal of the time with his eyes closed and his head back, almost musing aloud to himself, to an entirely hushed room of twelve hundred faculty, students, and staff in Kresge Auditorium, at the very heart of the MIT campus.*

George blew the house down with that speech. He was a great orator, but that speech turned out to be the most momentous political speech of his entire life, and the one that catapulted him into a

---

* Thirty-four years later, I was back in Kresge, where, in September 2003, the Mind and Life Institute, in collaboration with MIT's McGovern Brain Institute, held the first public dialogue between Western neuroscientists and psychologists and the Dalai Lama and Buddhist monks and scholars on the subject of investigating the mind from both the interior, first-person, meditative perspective, and from the outer, third-person, traditional scientific perspective in the hope of such conversations spurring new avenues of scientific research and understanding of the nature of the mind. The juxtaposition of these two events in my memory is richly poignant. George, who was long gone by that time, would have loved it.

much higher level of commitment to political activism for peace. The speech was printed in its entirety as a centerfold in the main section of the *Boston Globe* several days later (March 8, 1969) as part of the coverage and follow-up of the events at MIT. The printed version was so much in demand that the *Globe* reprinted another half-million copies of it as a stand-alone flyer for free distribution. Nothing like that had ever happened before, and nothing like it, as far as I know, has happened since.

I tell this story to give a sense of what tiny groups of people can do to set rotations in consciousness in motion that can grow larger than could be imagined. Every generation needs to come to its own view of what is actually going on in the world, and how to interface with what has been inherited and contribute its own energies and imagination to what is most worth preserving and what needs to be reconfigured to serve a larger purpose that may not have been perceived earlier. Every generation needs to make its own assessment of what it has inherited from its elders, and usually the reading of that legacy is not entirely pretty. Nevertheless, it needs to be described accurately or we will just sink more deeply into delusion and somnambulance, and thus perhaps cause even greater harm to unfold, including to ourselves. By our willingness to accurately name what is, we can take steps to lovingly perturb the organism, the system, the body politic in specific and hopefully wise ways, in the best spirit of patriotism and a free society, ways that may generate new lenses through which to see things and really apprehend them as they are, and thus give rise to new unthought-of options for dealing with age-old problems. It is not even so much the means that are most important, but the quality of mind and heart behind the means. There is no ignoring or eschewing or escaping the power of even a tiny bit of wisdom and sanity when it comes to shaping our interfaces with the world. But that power needs to be cultivated. Continually. Selflessly. Joyfully.

George Wald may have named what needed naming on that

particular day, at least in the minds and hearts of many of his listeners, but we need to do something similar for ourselves pretty much every day. Otherwise we may run the risk of losing touch with what we are actually doing on this planet. We can easily drift away from remembering how much the body politic depends on the agency of all of us, and how much our agency is based on our own inner development and understanding of who we are and how we are treating the world as well as on how the world is treating us; on what we are offering the world as well as what the world is offering us.

That process is timeless, the timelessness of awareness itself. Yet it needs to take place in time as well, virtually continuously, given the perpetual dis-ease and crisis of our species and our planet and our time. Imagination has a huge role to play here. Over time, we have the potential to recognize and grow into our truest and most authentic selves, each in our own way and according to our own heart. We have the potential to discern how much of our own actions or inactions may be driven by greed, hatred, delusion, or just plain inertia and ignorance, and to work consciously—again, to whatever degree it feels appropriate, both inwardly and outwardly—to *learn* our way out of our unwise and dukkha-deepening habits of seeing only what we want to see, and doing what we want to do without taking in the frequently harmful consequences of our choices. Instead, we can consciously opt for pathways that recognize the pain we inadvertently or purposefully cause each other in this world, and find ways to inhabit a greater silence and sense of security that are the cornerstone of seeing the other in oneself and thus, of peace. Our true crisis is one of consciousness. Our true liberation is in consciousness. Hmmmmm.

Many people at that time thought we had to fight a war in Vietnam to contain Communism—and that if we didn't, pretty soon, the proverbial "dominos" of that era would be falling everywhere and we would wind up communist ourselves. It turned out not to be such a good assessment of the situation. The disease wasn't really in

Vietnam, or at least not the disease we needed to concern ourselves with. It was in our way of seeing. It was in ourselves and in our fear. It still is.

The price tag for such misadventures is enormous, morally and monetarily, socially and spiritually. And we wonder why so many people around the globe at times perceive *us* as more of a threat to civilization than the obvious "bad guys," when our perception of ourselves seems to be that we mean so well and try so hard and do so many good and altruistic things, even in war. In our own minds at least, *we* are always the "good guys," even though in this era, the "guys" word now subsumes all genders. I guess it just boils down to the fact that as a species, we are still in our infancy in many ways, still learning, cliché that it may be, that it is easier to win a war than it is to nurture a lasting peace. Only now, it is not even clear what winning would look like. And war now seems to be endless. Perhaps we are really at war with ourselves. If so, perhaps we need to unilaterally declare and work toward a lasting peace. How about right now?

As we noted in the Foreword, the motto of the United States Air Force is: "Eternal vigilance is the price of freedom." It is so much more true than whatever ad agency thought it up might have suspected. That vigilance needs to be nurtured through mindfulness on every level, not just on the radar screen or at airport security. That freedom we hold so dear needs to be deeply appreciated and understood. If we want to be liberators, perhaps we might do well first to liberate ourselves from our own unawareness and endemic blindness through a kind and gentle, but, at the same time, fierce and firm inwardly directed vigilance.

# WAG THE DOG

In the uncannily prescient 1997 movie of that name, a fictitious admin-istration in the White House enlists a spin doctor and a Hollywood producer to fabricate a war with a Balkan country to distract voters from a presidential sex scandal. A totally concocted provocative event is broadcast repeatedly on television as breaking news. It does the trick, incensing and inflaming the citizenry and producing the justification for going to war. Never mind that the episode itself never happened.

Time and again we are seeing that some of our politicians are willing to say and do or go along with virtually *anything* to convince us of truths that just aren't so, maybe based on tiny episodes or events that meant something entirely different, or maybe on the basis of events that never happened at all. The infamous 1964 Gulf of Tonkin incident that occasioned our claiming that the North Vietnamese attacked one of our warships and led to ten years of carnage and dev-astation was just such an episode. From all reports, it never happened. There was no attack. Whether this phenomenon occurs as a product of Machiavellian conniving and cynical power-lust or simply from well-intentioned naïveté and mindlessness run amok in government is an open question, but whatever the underlying motive, it usually gets us to the same unfortunate place all the same.

It seems that nowadays, all politicians or pundits need to do is say something is blue and, even if it is obviously red, some fraction of the media will print that it is blue and enough people will believe it because they read it in the paper or saw it on the news so that it at least becomes a debatable point, as if it were true, and thus may be perceived by many as an outright assault on our country and therefore an occasion for righteous indignation and an overwhelming response to show we cannot be threatened, pushed around, and bullied. We are no longer held accountable for our claims. Anything is possible, no matter how implausible and unsupported by the evidence. In 2018, the president of the United States lies brazenly and apparently compulsively on a daily basis. But outright lying or more subtle dissimulation goes way back in time.

Perhaps red really *is* blue. Pick whatever instance you like. Perhaps there was a connection between Iraq and the attacks of September 11. As soon as it is said, even if the evidence marshaled for it was minimal or implausible, or for that matter totally fabricated, which it turned out to be, it takes on the qualities of the truth for many people, especially if it is then said over and over again, and within a context of fearmongering that exploits our understandable feelings of insecurity. "If we don't stop the terrorists in Iraq, we will be at their mercy at home with more attacks on innocent people, unthinkable attacks, even using weapons of mass destruction acquired from rogue states. Sounds plausible. Let's attack them before they attack us. Especially since we are the good guys, and the aggrieved party. Never mind stopping and analyzing the situation fully. Never mind what our allies and friends are saying. Things are different now. They are either with us or against us. Blue is red now, and those who say that, no, it is still blue, are not to be trusted. They are obviously unpatriotic. They don't care about the peril that freedom and democracy find themselves in." It is wag the dog, all over again.

And so our secretary of state lied bold-facedly at the UN. We won a "preemptive" war, or so we thought, ousted a monstrous and murderous dictator that nobody was sad to see go except his war criminal cronies, "liberated" the country, and wound up in a different kind of morass. Arguably, we restored life and purpose to Al Qaeda in the U.S. prisons in Iraq, and effectively filled the ranks of terrorist organizations worldwide, such as ISIS, for a decade with new recruits, based on our arrogance, our own abuses of power, and our need to be a force for good in our own eyes, whatever the cost, often for all the wrong reasons. This was more than a decade before Donald Trump.

Does distorting the truth ever make us any safer? George Orwell wrote *1984* as a cautionary tale of what can happen when we refuse to call a spade a spade when the moment requires it, and are thus hood-winked, or hoodwink ourselves into thinking that red is blue and blue is red, white is black and black is white, or, as he put it, "War is Peace/ Freedom is Slavery."

And it can hardly have escaped the notice of many that a quota-tion attributed to the Nazi General Hermann Goering, at the Nurem-berg War Trials following World War II, was widely circulated on the Internet in the wake of the preemptive invasion of Iraq, framing the wag-the-dog phenomenon in a terrifying way:

> "Naturally the common people don't want war, but after all, it is the leaders of a country who determine the policy, and it is always a simple matter to drag people along whether it is a democracy, or a fascist dictatorship, or a parliament, or a communist dictatorship. Voice or no voice, the people can always be brought to the bidding of the leaders. This is easy. All you have to do is tell them they are being attacked, and denounce the pacifists for lack of patriotism and exposing the country to danger. It works the same in every country."

It is bad enough to fall into red or blue, or black or white think-ing and the either-or, us-or-them judgments that stem reflexively from such distorted perception. But when we are asked so much of the time to accept that black is white or that red is blue, it pushes the boundaries of credulity, when we know that most situations are com-plex and often ambiguous, and require discernment and insight and a careful weighing of options and consequences against the backdrop of wisdom in order to deliver true security and promote wise action in the world. And yet, the evidence is all too plain that, given the right causes and conditions, manipulated by the right people under the right circumstances, using the right language and playing on our fears and prejudices, and encouraging us to ignore our capacity for clear seeing and for discerning what is so and to what degree it may be so, as a society we collectively fall time and again into mindlessness, caught up in spasms of madness that truly do threaten our well-being and even our integrity as a nation, and even as a species.

Might it not be time to wake up, and when it looks like the tail might be wagging the dog to say so, and refuse to be lulled or coerced into passivity and somnambulance and surrender our freedom, our liberty, and our common sense at the altar of mindlessness, fear, and manipulation? Might it not be past time for us to start paying attention to what is both inwardly and outwardly actually going on beneath the surface appearance of events, and not ignore the signs and symptoms of the underlying disease and its ultimate toxicity? Might it not be time to act appropriately based on the full range of our multiple intelligences, and not merely on suspect military intelligence filtered through minds that may have their own biased agendas and therefore may do anything *but* contribute to enhancing clarity and accuracy in assessing a complex situation? Might it not be just the right time for us to take responsibility as a nation and as individuals to "be all we can be," as the U.S. Army would have it? Or maybe it is way past that time, and we need to play serious catch up. Only time will tell.

# "I Don't Know What I Would Have Done Without My Practice!"

I am continually moved by the many people who come up to me in my travels, briefly recount one version or another of the full catastrophe occurring in their lives, and then say in so many words: "I don't know what I would have done without my practice." They are referring to their meditation practice, of course, and the various ways they have discovered to hold experience, any experience, which make both it and them come alive.

When we settle into awareness in the present moment, we invariably feel ourselves in intimate relationship with things as they are, however they are. Of course, we are in intimate relationship with them anyway, whether we know it or not. But without a more-than-conceptual knowing—without awareness—we are seriously handicapped in our ability to recognize, understand, acknowledge, and accept the actuality of our situation, especially when it is not to our liking. As a consequence, we may be seriously handicapped in our ability to act in ways that are both wise and kind and also useful, even healing. Unwise actions often merely compound difficult situations without our even knowing where the source of the increasing impediments lies. Actually, we are throwing obstacles out in front of us as we go forward.

Mindfulness is a gateway to restoring a degree of balance and clarity at the interface between the inner and outer worlds. It reminds us of how we might embody a greater degree of wisdom and perhaps even a modicum of compassion right here and right now; how we might embody, at least to some degree, freedom from affliction and emotional turmoil right in the midst of affliction and emotional turmoil, and without shutting ourselves off from them. As a practice, mindfulness has the capacity to calm the heart and focus and clarify the mind in any season of a life, even in the midst of the most horrific and tempestuous storms, without in the slightest disregarding or minimizing the anguish and the enormity of the suffering that may be involved and the need to go on in the face of huge and painful uncertainties.

And where do that wisdom and compassion come from? They come from inside you—they are part of your makeup, which you can come to embody in greater measure if you care to, just by keeping up the practice. And once you give yourself over to the ongoing moment-to-moment cultivation of mindfulness both formally and in everyday life in whatever modest ways you can manage, you may find that everything becomes your teacher—in other words, the world itself collaborates in offering up to us endless examples and sources of wisdom and compassion.

So again, just as a reminder that bears repeating many many times over, meditation is not what you think (see Book 1). It is not some kind of inward maneuver that shuts down thinking and suppresses feelings and papers things over with an artificial, saccharine, pretend "spiritual" calmness, although a lot of people think this about meditation when they don't practice, and sometimes even when they do. It is not about fixing or curing or arriving or attaining some special state. Mindfulness is not a state at all. It is a going beyond all states of mind, and all opinions, even all diagnoses. It is a way of being in relationship with experience in the only moment we ever get. It is a coming to rest in awareness itself, an awareness that can hold whatever is happening while it is happening, without pushing anything away, even if it is unpleasant or painful and we don't want it to be here, and without pursuing any experience and obsessing about it endlessly, even if it is extremely pleasant and we don't want it to go away. And as we have seen (Book 2) awareness is not something we have to acquire or develop. We are born with it, just as we are born with feet and hands. It is a core aspect of our being human. What the practice of meditation does develop is *access* to our capacity for awareness so that we can, metaphorically, take up residency in that spacious nonconceptual knowing quality of the human mind and allow it to become our default mode and help us to navigate the actuality of life unfolding moment by moment and day by day.

Meditation is really about freedom. As we have been discovering throughout all four books in this series, mindfulness is first and foremost a liberative practice. It is a way of being that puts us back in touch with the full dimensionality of our life and our intrinsic completeness, embodied right here, right now—wresting it from the jaws of unawareness and the habits of inattention and somnambulance that threaten to imprison us in ways that can be as painful, ultimately, as losing our outward freedoms. And one way it frees us is from continually making the same unwise decisions when the consequences of such are staring us right in the face and could be apprehended if only we would look and actually see.

For all these reasons, mindfulness can be a natural catalyst in deepening and broadening democracy, a democracy in which liberty is embodied not only in our rhetoric and in our laws and institutions and how they are implemented in practice, as critically important as that is, but also in our hard-earned wisdom as individual citizens, stemming from looking deeply into our true nature and experiencing it directly from inside, a wisdom that is embodied in our hearts and in our love for the interior landscapes of the mind and the heart and of the body as well. The more we become intimate with this landscape, the more familiar it is to us, the more we can participate effectively in society, and appreciate the beauty and unique potential of every single one of us. The more people come to know this terrain from the inside, the more we will all benefit from sharing in a distributive wisdom and goodwill of mutual regard that can translate into healthier communities and a healthier society, and a nation that knows its priorities and lives them in the world with authentic and unwavering reverence and respect.

That kind of liberty cannot know borders. If others are not free, then in a very real way, we cannot be completely free or at peace either, just as we cannot be completely healthy in an unhealthy world. But that does not mean that we are somehow divinely anointed to export our definition and view of freedom to other cultures. Far better to be grounded in and devote our energies to healing, to the valuing and restoring of wholeness at every level of society, to finding common human ground. This is the real waging of peace and of politics, the waging of wisdom in the world. This is potentially the deepest and most satisfying expression of our imagination and our strength, a source of real satisfaction, of happiness, of well-being. As a nation, and as a species, we now need our inner strengths to match or exceed our outward strengths. We need to grow into our wholeness. The alternatives are too horrific to contemplate. So maybe we should.

Perhaps a day will come when the president of the United States will turn toward her partner or husband, at the end of a long and trying day, and say: "Honey, I don't know what I would have done without my practice."

# The Suspension of Distraction

In the week following 9/11, an editor at the *Village Voice* was asked on NPR how he perceived the effect of the attack on the psyche of the city and its inhabitants. He characterized it as a "suspension of distraction." He had noticed that people were making eye contact with each other as never before, that they were communing silently with passing glances, taking in one another's faces. They did not seem to be absorbed in life's usual preoccupations and mind states. The inconceivable event, the horror of it, the huge loss of life, the evaporation of the city's two signature buildings, had plunged New Yorkers into wordless presence in the face of the enormity of what had occurred.

The suspension of distraction. A telling phrase. Its poignancy struck home as a hopeful signature of humanity's resilience, even wisdom, in a time of great wounding and grief.

The suspension of distraction. How amazing for a city and a society in which we are entrained into lives of virtually perpetual distraction, where everything is competing for our attention, assaulting our senses and our minds, and where we so often protect ourselves from the onslaught with distractions of our own, and in the process, forget what is most important to us, and even who we are and what we are doing.

I don't know how long the culture of distraction that New Yorkers are so practiced at was in abeyance, because certainly a return to the norm and the normal has to be a part of the healing process. But there was a lot to wake up to on that day. It revealed for sure that a fulminating dis-ease, up to that point unrecognized, ignored, and untreated, in spite of a series of highly significant warning signs, perhaps even *compounded* by our lack of understanding of interconnectedness, can find its way into the heart of our body politic and wreak untold suffering and damage.

We were also reminded in the most graphic of ways that everything is impermanent. Underscore *everything*. Of course we already knew this deep down. But in the daily conduct of our lives, we pretend to ourselves that we are immortal and that our creations last, and that life unfolds with a degree of reliability and certainty, and that the bad things only happen elsewhere, to other, more unfortunate people. One of the purposes of the social order in a peaceful, healthy society is to insure a high degree of relative certainty and safety for its inhabitants through the rule of law, backed up by effective law enforcement and an impartial judicial system, a common defense, a good health care system, and a sense of the possible through educational, economic, and creative opportunities. That at least is the ideal. In practice it is only an approximation that continually requires refining and deepening. Nevertheless, the law of impermanence is always at work, no matter how good or effective our institutions are or are not in any moment. Everything changes. Nothing remains the same for long. Things are fundamentally uncertain. In times of social strife and instability, the effects of this law seem magnified, and more unpredictable. That in itself can be terrifying.

September 11 showed us that even our great buildings are impermanent and can be vaporized in no time through human ignorance and malevolence. It reminded us that our lives, even in youth, even in health, even in peacetime, even in the midst of a great city in a great country are subject to the law of impermanence. At eight o'clock that morning, the enormous towers, which cast shadows over lower Manhattan and blocked out much of the sky, were there, as they had been since they were constructed in the 1960s. By 10:30 that morning, they were gone. For impermanence to reveal itself on such a massive scale, in peacetime, with such tragic loss of life and the robbery of countless hopes and dreams, parents and breadwinners, in virtually the blink of an eye, truly was unthinkable.

And just as what was left was a huge empty space, which was immediately hallowed by the enormity of the loss of life and by the selfless efforts of those who lived and died in the rescue efforts and those who contributed their psyches and their bodies to the clean-up, so the insubstantiality of what we hold as most tangible, most real was also poignantly revealed.

Yeats observed that "all things fall and are built again." But never have we collectively experienced in our own home—seared onto our retinas and into our brains through images and footage that words cannot capture, and breaking our hearts—that so much and so many could disappear so quickly. A certain innocence was lost that day. Part of it comes from waking up, not a bad thing, but in this case so cruelly revealing that form is emptiness.

Of course, Hiroshima and Nagasaki were also seared into our retinas, although not as the attacks were happening, and the destruction occurred even more rapidly, virtually instantaneously, and on a much vaster scale. But the mind also forgets rapidly. That was another era, before the ubiquity of television. Besides, we were at war and "they" were the enemy. "They" had attacked us, without warning.

Yes, and "they," the people of Hiroshima and Nagasaki, were civilians going about their lives, merely people living in cities. They too suffered at the hands of their leaders who were pursuing their own ideas of imperial grandeur and a sense of being right, which is always an unexamined "fact" when it is your tribe. True, they were part of the tribe that chose to aggress, but those women and children and the elderly and the laborers had as little to do with Pearl Harbor or the rape of Nanking as the stock traders at Cantor Fitzgerald had to do with grievances in the Muslim world.

Perhaps it is time for us to realize once and for all that there is only one tribe here, that there is only one planet that we all inhabit, one living body suffering from inflammations and infections that are crying out to be soothed, salved, and healed. Our response cannot simply be to beef up the immune system of our country or our network of allies, although that is important within a larger framework of true intelligence (every pun intended). But we are our own enemy here. If we keep distracting ourselves from the ways in which our actions generate hatred and contempt, if we say one thing but do another, profess democratic ideals but then force issues because we have enough power to do so, if we persist in thinking that we can market ourselves to the world rather than embodying our deepest principles in our policies and actions, we will not be able to name, face, or heal the source of the worldwide dis-ease we are individually and collectively suffering from. Perhaps it is time for us as a people and as a nation to linger collectively in the purposeful suspension of distraction and re-examine how we treat and understand each other, and how we hold our own suffering so that it leads to wisdom, not greater ignorance and even more suffering for ourselves and for others.

Perhaps it is time to make suspension of distraction a way of life. Imagine how healthy it might be for us personally, and for the world at large. We might truly come to know peace because we would be peaceful. Not naïve, not weak, not powerless but truly powerful, peace-embodying and peace-appreciating, in our true strength, in our true wisdom.

Why on Earth not?

# Moments of Silence

Gathered at the place that has come to be known as Ground Zero in New York City, on September 11, 2002, at precisely the moment the first plane went into the north tower of the World Trade Center one year before, the family members of those who died and those who survived, along with sundry dignitaries, onlookers, and those for whom it was a solemn pilgrimage, were asked to observe a moment of silence.

Driving down the highway in Massachusetts, I participated in that silence via the radio as no doubt millions of others did across the country and around the world. Everybody knew what to do. We were not given instructions. No one suggested how to feel, or what to feel, or how to deal with our thoughts and emotions. It would have been absurd and disrespectful and wholly inappropriate. It would never have crossed the organizers' minds to include any instructions for how to hold a moment like that. It just wasn't and isn't necessary in such circumstances.

Everybody already knows what a moment of silence is. We were all one in that silence, even as we were each with our own unique thoughts, our own unique emotions, our own sense of purpose and loss, whatever our relationship to the event was. And for each of us, as we know because it is so obvious, it is totally different.

When an event stirs great sadness and grief in us, after the wailing and the tears and the tearing of our hair, there comes a time when we have to fall silent. It is even beyond prayer. Prayers, which are also offered up at such moments, do not substitute for silence. Silence is the ultimate prayer.

We call a moment of silence an observance. How appropriate. It is a falling into the present moment with awareness and an openness of heart that allows for all our feelings, speakable and unspeakable, reconciling and vengeful, hopeful and despairing to just be here. It is a moment of pure being. It is also a nod to something deep within ourselves that we touch only briefly and then shy away from, perhaps out of discomfort or pure unfamiliarity. It is a bearing witness. In that bearing witness, we not only bear our burden better, but we demonstrate that we are larger than it is, that we have the capacity to hold it, to honor it, and to make a context for it and for ourselves, and so grow beyond it without ever forgetting.

In reflecting on my experience later that day, I began imagining what it would have been like if instead of a moment of silence, we had been asked to observe five minutes of silence, or ten, or even an hour. Would we have still known how to be in the face of the enormity and barbarity and senselessness of it all? We might expect that of a Desmond Tutu or a Dalai Lama, a Mother Theresa or a Martin Luther King. But what about us regular folk? Would we be able to sustain an awareness of the rupture of our hearts? Could we be still? What if we didn't know how long it would last? Could we still inhabit that place in ourselves from which observing and bearing witness happen? After all, we don't "make" it happen. Could we still inhabit that place in us which is speechless, which bears witness to the full extent of what has come to pass, including the unknowableness of what it will mean for the future? Could we still inhabit that place of what in this moment just is, with no boundaries anymore between past, present, and future, all of which are alive for us now in what is known and what remains unknown? And wouldn't such a silence work on us, stretch us, challenge us, grow us, change us, heal us? I think so.

Surely a memorial service is not just about memory. It is a

confluence of memory and now. It is about honoring the dead and the harmed and the heroic in the present moment, which is always now, for now is ironically, mysteriously, the only actuality that endures.

Even the briefest moment of silence is both a way of coming into the present and a way of moving on. It offers closure, or at least, the marking of a watershed moment. We know that closure may come to us in some ways, but in other ways we know it never will. This led me to wonder whether we could observe a moment of silence not only in memory (as in memorial) of what had come to pass, but of what is passing as it comes to pass. Could we meet anger, including our own anger, with silence as it is arising, and bear witness to it in the same way? Could we meet disbelief, grief, fear, despair, hatred, the impulse for vengeance, with moments of silence?

It seems to me that we already have this capacity within us. Otherwise, we would not make use of moments of silence in our public ceremonies and instinctively, intuitively, wisely know how to be in them, which is always just as we are, with awareness, doing nothing, observing and thereby embracing the fullness of what is…for now, beyond any doing.

For now.

# The Ascendancy of the Mindful

The former *New York Times* war correspondent Chris Hedges calls patriotism, in its conventional guise, a "thinly veiled form of collective self-worship." He points out that in the twentieth century alone, over 62 million civilians perished in war, nearly 20 million more than the 43 million military personnel killed. When there is talk of bloodletting, it is all too literal.

And for what? Aren't the events leading to war so often the result of blind attachment to deranged and increasingly self-intoxicating views that become perpetrated, as Hedges points out, as national myths that cannot be gainsaid during the spasm of conflict and the time leading up to it, but which afterward everyone on both sides can agree appear as madness, as folly, as potentially preventable, as an endemic disease of cataclysmic proportions?

Consider overall German behavior in World War II. Systematic aggression, genocide, murder, and mayhem, bureaucratized on an unprecedented scale, orchestrated as if they were accountants keeping track of inventories, as if they had no moral scruples or human sensibilities. Was it the "evil" of all Germans, or merely their understandable timidity and retreat into denial and grotesque compartmentalization and rationalization in the face of what began as a violent and ruthless minority perpetrating a myth many Germans in that day somehow perhaps wanted to believe, a myth of their own greatness and the inferiority of others to the point of dehumanizing them and systematically trying to eradicate them that secretly resonated in and warped their very humanity, perhaps, in some cases at least, despite their instincts and better judgment?

Now they are our friends. Only three generations have passed. They are us now, and it certainly feels that way when I teach there and spend time with wonderful friends and colleagues. The Marshall Plan restored Germany as a prosperous society after the cataclysm. It was an act of huge moral wisdom and economic foresight on the part of America. The disease of Nazism is past only because it was met head-on. Perhaps there is now an immunity of sorts in their society or in others, but for how long? The United States accumulated huge goodwill in the world in the aftermath of that war, by our sacrifice, and by our generosity and wisdom. But that goodwill of another generation and another era is long gone. Goodwill can be squandered if we drift too far from our intrinsic goodness, and remain blind to our own drifting, soothed and lulled to sleep by our own unexamined rhetoric, forgetting that things change, and forgetting just how much we need to pay attention and understand how things are now.

Just like other viruses, the viruses of fear and hatred have ways of going latent for longer than our memories, then reinfecting us with the same thinly veiled platitudes, half-truths, otherings of all kinds such as racism, anti-Semitism, homophobia, "the enemy," "them" as opposed to "us," the intruders, the poor, the immigrants, those who don't belong and aren't welcome, and forms of pompous righteousness that call for blood when wisdom calls for reason, kindness, diplomacy, and patience in most cases, and perhaps, in some cases, such as when genocide is being perpetrated, quick, nuanced, measured, skillful, and tough international police or military action, all the while keeping the bigger picture, the whole in mind.

We will need to cultivate wisdom and mindfulness as if our very lives depended on it, and our integrity, keeping our priorities straight, if we have even the remotest hope of not succumbing to the lowest common denominator of our historical karma—to apply a massive military approach first when, in this era, a medical, diplomatic, even surgical one would be more appropriate. Conflicts are inward as much as they are outward. With wisdom more intentionally cultivated in politics and diplomacy, many crises can be averted, headed off before they grow to the point where the scourge of ignorance masquerading as evil can only be met by military might to preserve or restore freedom and happiness, and presumably, new market opportunities. For such wisdom to prevail, perhaps we need to develop our inner skills to match the sophistication of our weaponry and combat training. For that, perhaps there could and should be more moments of silence, genuine silence and reflection in the House and the Senate, in the Pentagon and in the White House, everywhere.

I was at the Library of Congress when the Vietnamese Zen Master, mindfulness teacher, poet, and peace activist Thich Nhat Hanh gave a talk on mindfulness one evening for members of Congress and their families. He started out by holding up both arms and saying something like, "With this arm [indicating the right one] I write poetry, with this other arm, I don't. But does that mean that one arm is less than the other? They are both part of my body, and I need to honor them both." He was referring to different countries and people with differing viewpoints, customs, and beliefs, all part of this one world, just like both arms, however different, are part of his one body. That talk introduced a mindfulness retreat offered just for members of Congress and their families. Twelve representatives attended at least parts of it. Nothing like it had ever happened before. And very little of note came of it, at least as far as we know.

Still, one never knows what happens to the seeds one plants. Some remain latent for long stretches of time before sprouting up. Life is messy most of the time, and complicated. We need to recognize that and welcome it rather than be deterred or discouraged by what seem like overwhelming obstacles to transformation. That Congressional weekend may not have been a major turning point. Or perhaps it was and we will only know in retrospect far down the road. Perhaps Thich Nhat Hanh's visit and the Dalai Lama's periodic appearances in Washington have already planted seeds of mindfulness that can be watered as a real and commonsensical choice in the lives of those whose job it is to guard the common good, the commonweal. Perhaps these seeds will germinate and grow as people come to understand their value—way beyond the Buddhism that it is so easy to think of them as and so easy for some to dismiss them as when the exponents are monastics from other cultures—and their relevance as balm and medicine for our anguished hearts and agitated minds, as windows on the inner and outer worlds through which to see with eyes of wholeness. In that seeing, that realizing, we finally do come to our senses, not as an end it itself but as a way of being, as a new beginning, a reaffirmation of our wholeness as human beings, of our potential for living wisely and for loving what is here for us to love, in the midst of the messiness. Perhaps it will become more apparent to us as these seeds sprout and flower in our society to an increasing degree, that they are not about somebody else—they are always about us, about me, about you, about us humans, *Homo sapiens sapiens*, the species that is aware and is aware that it is aware. Time to live our way into that name. Or way past time.

The poet John Donne said "never send to know for whom the bell tolls; it tolls for thee." The bell Donne was referring to is the funeral bell, the bell that reminds us of our brief sojourn in this world. But there is another bell, the bell of mindfulness, that tolls in each moment as well, or can, if we are paying attention, inviting us to rediscover and come back to our senses in this very moment, reminding us that it is possible to wake up to our lives now, while we have them to live. The bell of mindfulness tolls for thee as well. It tolls for all of us. It tolls in celebration of life and what might be, were we to hear it in its fullness, were we to wake up.

For those whose responsibility it is for a time to tend the well-being of the body politic by creating and refining laws out of a collective wisdom we can trust because they are us and we are them and we all know it, and for those chosen for a brief time to steer the ship of state, because they too are us and we are them and they know it, and for those whose job it is to uphold the laws that govern how we conduct our lives, an intimate understanding and respect for the underlying lawfulness of things, for the beauty of the delicate balance that we are in being alive, for what we have been calling universal dharma, or tao, or homeostasis, or harmony, or peace, or whatever other name you chose to give it, is indispensable. That cherishing, that remembering, that honoring, even in the face of the knottiest problems and their endemic resistance to change or reconciliation, may allow us all to flourish and gradually heal our wounds in a world that also flourishes in an ever-changing dynamical unfolding that prioritizes ethical behavior, non-harming, benevolence, truth, and the wisdom of both knowing and not knowing, and knowing when we don't know, in the face of constant change. In this way, we can individually and collectively continually nurture the emergence of what is truly possible for ourselves and for the generations to follow, for all sentient beings, and for this planet we call home.

Hey, stranger things have happened. We human beings are amazingly unpredictable, and full of surprises. Ultimately, perhaps we will surprise even ourselves.

> Power properly understood is nothing but the ability to achieve purpose. And one of the great problems of history is that the concepts of love and power have usually been contrasted as opposites—polar opposites—so that love is identified with a resignation of power, and power with a denial of love.
>
> We've got to get this thing right. What is needed is a realization that power without love is reckless and abusive, and love without power is sentimental and anemic. Power at its best is love implementing the demands of justice, and justice at its best is power correcting everything that stands against love. It is precisely this collision of immoral power with powerless morality which constitutes the major crisis of our time.
>
> MARTIN LUTHER KING, JR., 1967, in his last
> address as president of the Southern Christian
> Leadership Conference

# PART 2

# LET THE BEAUTY WE LOVE BE WHAT WE DO

———————

*Today like every other day*
*We wake up empty and scared.*
*Don't open the door of your study*
*And begin reading.*
*Take down a musical instrument.*
*Let the beauty we love be what we do.*
*There are hundreds of ways to kneel*
*And kiss the earth.*

RUMI

# Different Ways of Knowing
## Make Us Wiser

Across the span of nine hundred years, Rumi is evoking reverence for the moment and how easily it can be missed if, in the face of our endemic discomfort and dis-ease, we persist out of habit in opening the door of our study and begin reading (and thinking) when we might, alternatively, "take down a musical instrument," the closest at hand being our own living body, and let the beauty we love, if we can be in touch with it, reveal itself in the many different ways we might carry ourselves in this moment, here and now. This is nothing less than an exhortation to practice being truly in touch with what is most fundamental, most important, and a nod to there being no singular one right way to go about it.

Reverence arises when faced with the incomprehensible. And by incomprehensible, I don't mean that something cannot be understood. I mean that whatever it is that we are attending to can be understood in many different ways. And yet, when all is said and done and we have come to the end of all our thoughts, no matter how brilliant, imaginative, and informed, all our logic no matter how grounded in reason, all our studies, there is a residue of feeling that goes beyond thought altogether, as when transported by some marvelous strains of music, or when struck by the artistry of a great painting, or the miracle of a chrysalis, or of a beam of sunlight through redwoods. A feeling of awe arises that transcends mere explanation. The actuality—whatever it is—hovers in the mystery of its undeniable phenomenological presence in relationship to our senses, including the non-conceptual, apprehending, knowing mind. I am speaking of the mystery of the very existence of an event or object, its "isness" as a phenomenon, its links with all other phenomena, all that has ever been, its numinous and luminous isness. In the case of a work of art, even the artist can't really articulate fully how it came about.

We don't have words for such numinous and luminous feelings, and often forget how prevalent they are in our experience. We can easily become inured to them and cease noticing that we even have such feelings or are capable of having them, so caught up we can be in a certain way of knowing to the exclusion of others. We can lose the reverence even when the wonder is incontrovertibly before us in every moment, in nature, in animals and plants, in mountains and rivers, valleys and vistas, even as we carry great cause for such reverence in our very being, in our own nature, in our very bones, in our very cells, in our being alive. We are so caught up in our habits of limited awareness or frank unawareness—mindlessness we could call it—that we can miss even the blue sky or the fragrance of a rose, the trilling of the lark or the wind on our skin, the ground beneath our feet or the smile of a baby's delight.

Having no words for this domain of relationality, we tend to fall back on the mechanical, which includes a lot of machine language, in an attempt to convince ourselves that we do understand. In fact, the dominant vocabulary for thinking about biology, about living organisms, and about the brain and the body and even the mind is machine language, machine imagery, machine analogies, and as we understand machines better and can make more extraordinary machines, our machine language and images get more and more refined, and perhaps even more and more convincing. And that now includes digital machines and soon, quantum machines, i.e. computers, and the algorithms that run them.

It is not uncommon for biologists to describe the fundamental unit of life, the cell, as a factory, filled with machinery and having characteristic inputs, outputs, control systems, functions that have, through evolving via natural selection over billions of years, given rise to all the complex structures and forms, the "machinery," that so effectively and so elegantly carries out those functions. The analogy works and is quite satisfying as far as it goes. Cells do function as very small factories, and here is where the awe comes in. They are nano-factories, working at the atomic and molecular level and right above it, with macromolecular structures, the whole of it seemingly designed and constructed by itself based on blueprints contained in its DNA and in its own structure, turning on and shutting off genes in various ways depending on the functions the cell "needs" to per-form (here we get into anthropomorphizing) and the fact that it can grow and reproduce. Each cell contains its own specialized structures and component machinery: ribosomes and endoplasmic reticulum for synthesizing proteins; the cell membrane and its ion channels and receptor-molecule-docking-stations for regulating bidirectional traffic between the interior of the cell and its environment, includ-ing other cells near and far; microtubules for structural scaffolding, movement, and transport within the cell; mitochondria that serve as power plants for the cell and seem to be tiny vestigial cells themselves, with their own DNA that took up residency billions of years ago within nucleated cells, and are present in numbers ranging from just a few to over ten thousand per cell, depending on the energy needs of the cell type. All this is a part of pretty much each cell in our body, with some specialized exceptions, like red blood cells. And keep in mind that this is not some mere abstraction. We know that these structures and many others are functioning constantly, in this and in every moment within our bodies, at the most minute molecular levels to keep us alive and breathing—it is what keeps our heart beating and allows us to see and feel and, somehow, even think.

And let's not forget, of course, that our cells are functioning in and as a society, a society of trillions of other cells in our one body, cells that they are related to through birth and through being part of a larger organism, and also through being part of the living world in which all organisms, great and small, share the same genetic code and the same machinery for reading it and building cells and sustaining themselves and reproducing. There are many many variations on a very few basic themes in living organisms on this planet at least, and cells are necessary for all of it to unfold.

Just think for a moment (how this society of cells manages to do that is an utter mystery) that we each grew from just one cell into, by common estimates, perhaps a hundred trillion cells, that is, 100,000,000,000,000 (here is where some math comes in handy for a convenient shorthand for conceptualizing and writing down such inconceivably large numbers, which very rapidly go beyond our sensory-based experience as the orders of magnitude mount: $10^2$ (one hundred) $\times 10^{12}$ (one trillion) $= 10^{14}$ (one hundred trillion)). Think for a moment that out of that one cell came all the different cells that make up your body and all the different structures that are made up of those cells: bone, muscle, skin, liver, heart, nerves, glands, even the "specialized" structures within the eyes, the ears, the nose, the tongue that allow us to sense light and sound and odor and taste and touch. It is mind-boggling, as is even how we move an arm or finger under volition. What is volition anyway, and where and how does it originate?

Just consider that inside your body, there are by some estimates a total of 67 billion miles of DNA threads, only two nanometers ($2 \times 10^{-9}$ meters) wide* and that the DNA doesn't just sit there but is constantly opening and closing and being read and repaired as it directs the ongoing functioning of the cell. And all that DNA fits, snugly compartmentalized into the tiniest of spaces inside the nuclei of our cells, residing within even more complex chromosomes that facilitate their genes being read according to the type of cell; and when it comes time to divide into two cells, the replication of themselves.

It is an unbelievable architectural achievement. Every aspect of the very design of living systems is literally incredible, not to be believed, far more sophisticated and miniature in scale than the most

---

* https://publications.nigms.nih.gov/insidelifescience/genetics-numbers.html

elaborate computer or machine we have ever developed. And consider that *each* neuron among the estimated 86 billion neurons in the human brain and central nervous system (to say nothing of approximately the same number of glial cells in the brain whose functions and "purpose" we only dimly understand) has over one thousand branching fingers (dendrites) that receive impulses from other nerve cells, which are reaching out to touch and nudge and amplify and temper its goings-on and that of its neighbors near and far through their own axons and dendrites. And, most mind-blowing of all, nowhere will you find a "you" in there, in any of the cells, in any of the parts.

What is more, each one of our neurons has numerous neurotransmitter receptor molecules embedded in the cell membrane at the synaptic junctions on its surface. These receptors are made up of protein molecules assembled together so that they open in response to specific chemical messengers (neurotransmitters) but remain closed otherwise, creating selective channels in the enveloping cell membrane that allow for changes in the state of the cell in response to changing conditions. At any and every level, the human body—and, veritably, every living organism—is truly a *universe* of unimagined complexity and also simplicity and elegance in its unity of functioning, in its wholeness, its very being.

And don't forget, we are talking about "you," not some far-out science fiction story about another galaxy and some other time.

And yet such ways of speaking of architecture and mechanism, of machines and factories, whether molecular or supra-molecular, are limited and limiting, even in their beautiful and partial truth.

What is left out are other ways we have of knowing who and what we are, ways that go way beyond our flair for logic, information flow, and thinking. For our mechanical descriptions and machine metaphors tend to leave out the reverence, the awe, the miracle of it all, the very isness of it. Those mechanistic descriptions leave out all that doesn't exactly get explained away no matter how much we know in our heads. They leave out *experience* and the mystery of *experiencing*. They leave out sentience. As reliable and impressive and as useful as many of our analytical and mechanistic ways of knowing about the world are, they tend to ignore the fact that there are always both smaller and larger areas that we do not understand, some that could only be known from a higher order, whole systems perspective, and complex enough so that perhaps they cannot be known completely, such as how the universe or our brains are (if I say "built" or "function" then I am in machine language already).

So at any one time, we are in the dark as well as in the light, endarkened as well as enlightened and illuminated, no matter how sophisticated our models and our explanations are. We suffer a certain deprivation and denaturation if we ignore these other ways we have of sensing, feeling, knowing and exploring our inner and outer landscapes. And we suffer as well if we fail to explore and become intimate with the boundaries of our knowing, the whole domain of our not knowing.

Of course we all know this. The clichéd example is selfless love. There is just no way to explain it or even describe it that does it justice. Poetry does better than neuroscience in this regard, but poetry and neuroscience are complementary, orthogonal ways of knowing. So both, and many other descriptions as well can be germane and illuminating, and pertain at the same time. Is what the poets know any less "real" than what science "knows"? I don't think so. Homer's view was every bit as true as Pythagoras's, and Homer was dealing with far more complex matters. That is not to denigrate Pythagoras in the slightest. His genius was of another sort, the first human really to delve into the nature of numbers and their relationships to each other, a feat of simultaneous abstraction and utter concreteness (what could be more concrete than a right triangle?), and who founded a mystical school to protect and revere that world and pursue its exploration as a sacred act.

But Homer was no slouch, and, as elucidated by Elaine Scarry in *Dreaming by the Book,* could use words to evoke with mind-bending skill the flight of a spear by describing the trajectory of its shadow, quite a squaring of the hypotenuse in its own right. And that is only one minor example. Some scholars have argued that the *Odyssey* and the *Iliad* contain all the important themes within Western civilization elaborated in Homer's wake.

Once we do "know" that the sum of the squares of the lengths of the two sides of a right triangle is equal to the square of the hypotenuse, we are extremely close to pure abstraction, a marvelous and mysterious feature of the domain we call *mind*. The greatest conundrum in mathematics for over three hundred years was Fermat's last theorem, which simply took the Pythagorean formula $a^2 + b^2 = c^2$ and upped the ante by upping the exponent, claiming that for all $a^n + b^n = c^n$, even the seemingly simplest case of $n = 3$, just one more than 2 (!), there exist no whole number solutions. Proving it was the holy grail of mathematics, and many great mathematicians failed in spite of heroic attempts—that is until it was finally proven by a superhuman feat of thought and motivation by Andrew Wiles, who, from the age of ten, devoted his life to seeking a solution to Fermat's challenge, and, after eight years of effort in secret, while pretending he was working on something else, but still, at the end, and importantly, with a little help from his friends, came up with the final proof in 1995.

We might wonder whether the world of mathematics is even real, in the concrete sense, given that it is so abstract. Yes, we know that numbers are for counting things, or heaps of things. But what about zero? What about the absence of things? The pile of no things of a certain kind? Or the absence of numbers in certain columns of numbers, what we call "place-holders"? What about the concept of "number" independent of things to be counted all together? Is this even meaningful? What about the fact that all numbers can be generated from zero and one, so just these two somehow have all of mathematics related to numbers latent within them, if we throw in a few axioms about how they operate together. And they also give us binary code and thus Turing machines made real, and thus computers, big data, algorithms, and the Mandelbrot set, among other marvels.

It is not so far-fetched to ask if mathematics is a property of the universe, or whether it is independent of any physical universe. Or is it a fabrication of the human mind, each mathematically inclined mind contributing to revealing some feature of the elephant without ever knowing the whole of it? Is there a mathematical sense? And if there is, what is it that is sensed, and who or what is doing the sensing? Why does mathematics lie behind the physical universe, as it appears it does? Why do physicists find that mathematics helps them to understand phenomena, that even abstractions like complex numbers, "discovered" centuries ago and that aren't really "real," based as they are on the square root of minus 1, are absolutely necessary, it seems, to accurately describe quantum phenomena only discovered in the past hundred years?

Mathematics is based only on logical proof, built up ever so cautiously from a very small number of starting axioms. When once something is proven, it is proven forever, and its "reality" is firmly established, even if it is in the nth dimension that our visual minds will never be able to imagine or know or sense, other than through the math itself.

Here, only mathematicians understand, and only within the narrow bands of their own specialties, I am told. In many ways, they function as a priesthood unto themselves, speaking a language that not even scientists understand, or sympathize with in many cases. Yet they tap "worlds" that are now absolutely critical for protecting information transfer in a digital age through cryptography, and to understanding the architecture of nature at the most minute level. Are these worlds creations of the human mind or are they discovered truths that transcend time and space and all physical realities, no matter how they are described? From the outside, mathematics has the feeling of a pristine universe of its own, mysterious, and self-consistent, and yet, always ultimately not completely knowable because of Kurt Gödel's incompleteness theorem, somewhat akin to the Heisenberg uncertainty principle in quantum physics.

When we do not limit ourselves to one way of knowing, or one vocabulary, or one set of lenses through which to look, when we purposefully expand our horizon of inquiry and curiosity, we can take delight in all the various ways we have of knowing something. We also have a chance to recognize the mystery of what is not known conceptually but sensed, felt, intuited, attended to by the confluence of all our senses in direct unfragmented experience, not excluding anything, even our concepts and what they reveal in any moment, all summing to an ongoing exchange with what is larger than we are and that is nothing other than us as well. Every one of our mysterious and miraculous senses, including mind, is a way of knowing the world and a way of knowing ourselves.

We are larger than any one way of knowing, and can enjoy all of them as different, incomplete, and complementary modes for appreciating what is and for *participating* in what is with gusto and delight for the moments—timeless and yet fleeting—that we are here for. We can always come back to and rest in not knowing as well as in knowing, delighting in the beauty of form and function as well as in their mystery and impersonal, deeply interconnected non-self nature on any and every level that the senses and the mind, our instruments and our instincts, our meditation practice, and our efforts and longing to understand deliver to us in any moment.

# On the Doorstep: Karma Meets Dharma—A Quantum Leap for *Homo Sapiens Sapiens*

It is astonishing how much good human beings have brought into the world.

It is astonishing how much harm human beings have inflicted on the world.

And in such a short time, too.

Barely twelve thousand years, say four hundred to six hundred generations (depending on how long we consider a generation to be) since the end of the last Ice Age and the dawn of history and what we call civilization, have given us the beauty and ingenuity of the sciences and the arts of all human cultures. A mere four to six hundred generations to produce the marvels and diverse expressions of agriculture, astronomy, and medicine, architecture and democracy with all their evolving wisdoms—and actually, of history *per se*, since recorded history doesn't begin until around 5000 to 2000 BCE in Sumaria, Egypt, and China, more like between two hundred fifty to one hundred fifty generations ago. That is actually very little time by biological standards. And even if you decide to go back further, to the dawn of *Homo sapiens*, say one hundred thousand years, or five thousand generations, or even further, in comparison to any geological measure of time, it has all unfolded virtually instantly, in the top few inches of the Grand Canyon's time card. From the perspective of cosmological time, the unfolding of human life has been even briefer, infinitesimally brief, minuscule against the backdrop of an almost unthinkably large infinitude of space and time birthed with the universe we inhabit, which by current measures is about 13.7 billion years old. And yet we can think of it, look both out into space and back in time (and looking out *is* looking back) and ponder that expanse of space and of time, and the mystery of our presence and our awareness here within it. Our mind in some amazing way can know and contain its infinitude.

We are one precocious species! We are capable of self-reflection, self-exploration, self-inquiry. And as far as we know, we are the only species that is so endowed, although we need to be mindful of being prone to a certain species chauvinism. Other species have their own intelligences that are in all likelihood equally extraordinary in their own ways, whether it be great apes or elephants or dolphins or birds or bees, dragonflies or worms, or even plants, to name just a few universes we don't understand and maybe can't in their fullness. They all have their own communities and ways of communing and communicating, as do we. But we humans seem capable of virtually limitless creativity, at least in some domains, and of translating those creative energies into tangible products. Imagine. We can manifest abstract mathematics and poetry out of living, throbbing, pulsating tissue. How on earth does that happen? Both math and poetry involve discovery and exploration in virtual worlds, in some ways existent, in some ways non-existent, worlds that take arduous effort to give birth to, wrestle with, and come to know. Amazing, when you think of it. Our capacity to know and to do, to make things and think, and look behind the appearance of things to some larger lawfulness sometimes seems staggeringly limitless.

As a species, we are named for our knowing, not our doing. In English the very term "human being" points directly at being, at awareness, at sentience. We do not, after all, call ourselves *human doings*, and for good reason, since our doing comes out of something larger that we intuitively know as being.

Yet we are capable as well of huge self-delusion, of mis-apprehending the whole of things, and at times, of mis-taking folly—especially our own—for wisdom. As we have seen over and over again, we *Homo sapiens* are capable of huge cruelty when we are most afraid and most deluded. Ironically, when we erupt out of fear and delusion, it is often under the banner of a greater good, usually our own, and in the name of a greater God, no surprise that it just happens to be our own as well. And it is usually at the expense of others not of our tribe. Or, when it is against others who we do not think of as mattering because we are thinking only of ourselves, if we are thinking at all, our behavior can be merely criminal rather than genocidal.

In six hundred generations or less, starting from small isolated communities, humans have explored the whole planet and populated much of it, generated diverse cultures, engaged in nigh-global commerce, and yet have managed to live episodically in fear, envy, or contempt of each other to such a degree that, now as ever-more-populous nations and even larger self-identifying groups, often religious in appearance, we have used our ingenuity to be perpetually at war with those by whom we feel threatened, or whose land or resources we covet. Our propensity for conflict has become a growing prescription for disaster. It has produced a wake of human suffering across those twelve-thousand-plus years, even as it has brought us to this day.

At this moment, our inheritance is truly a mixed blessing. Even as Charles Dickens characterized his time and that of the French Revolution, "It was the best of times, it was the worst of times...," so it is today. We have the beautiful, and we have the awful. We have the quintessential pinnacles of extraordinary cultures, and we have the detritus and destruction our seemingly innate bellicosity and belligerence have also wrought. If our inheritance is a mixed blessing, it is perhaps relevant to note that the word "blessing" already encodes this dilemma, carrying within it as it does the French word *blessure*, which means wound, as well as the meaning of benediction. Perhaps being so vulnerable and susceptible to wounding, we can grow into greater knowing, into our birthright, our namesake as a species, ultimately only through experiencing and accepting that woundedness and finding ways to honor it rather than to seal it off from our consciousness through the fear and anger that so often mask it, which only leads us to be endlessly propelled and conditioned by it.

Genetically speaking, we are one people. The two most seemingly different people in the world are virtually identical from the point of their genes.* At most, about one in a thousand nucleotides in our DNA are different between the blackest and the whitest, the tallest and the shortest of us. We are 99.9 percent the same. We are one tribe, one family, but have yet to recognize it. We humans are all intimately interconnected. How we treat each other matters to the health and well-being, perhaps even the survival, of us all as a species, not in some vague future, but in this very moment.

Of course, different cultures have vastly different ideas about interconnectedness and relationality. But twelve thousand years ago and earlier, those differences and animosities may not have mattered much for the well-being of the planet or the survival of the species, to say nothing of civilization and culture. Human groups lived separately from each other, each mostly intent on eating, sleeping, procreating, and surviving. Whatever they did, they were so much a part of the natural world and so much fewer in number than now that their lives and even their conflicts were relatively contained. Our late ancestors clearly had rich interior lives, as evidenced by their elaborate cave paintings and figurines, dating far back into Paleolithic times. Their art was extraordinary and their technology to ensure that it would endure equally so. Apparently even living in caves, the impulse to paint and celebrate the mystery of being alive in the vastness of nature, to affirm their experience of it, was unstoppable.

Twelve thousand years later, we are all crowded together on this planet as never before, our numbers increasing exponentially, as natural

---

* Eric Lander. Talk presented at the Mind and Life Institute Dialogue X: "The Nature of Mind, the Nature of Life," with His Holiness, the Dalai Lama, Dharamsala, India, October 2002. See Luisi, Pier Luig with Z. Houshmand, *Mind and Life: Discussions with the Dalai Lama on the Nature of Reality,* Columbia University Press, New York, 2008.

resources become ever scarcer. There are currents of continued hatred, animosity, and distrust among different cultures, even as we reach to transcend what we have always thought of as our blood ties and marriage to ancestral plots of land. The United Nations is one attempt to recognize that underlying unity we all share in, and to find peaceful ways to reconcile our differences. It is a noble effort, in its infancy, whatever it matures into, as are we and the nation-states we inhabit, for that matter.

To grow into ourselves fully as a species and as nations among nations, however long the concept and institution of "nation" is going to last, it seems time to recognize that we have gotten to this point in human history through a great deal of plunder and pillaging in addition to via our intrinsic goodness. We have all arrived here with the merciless subjugation of other peoples' land and living spaces in our past, always sanitized in the history books to sound like progress and the emergence of the inevitable. People accommodated, or didn't. Whole civilizations were decimated by pathogens they had no defenses against, subjugated, or put to the sword, in Yeats' phrase. This happened time and time again throughout history.

We know that America has the undeniable facts of genocide and hundreds of years of the enslavement of people in its past. And we know that it carries the enduring legacies of these atrocities right into to the present day. Why are we so intent on downplaying this history, or ignoring it completely? Obviously, because it hurts to look at and to see ourselves in it. Europeans wanted this world for themselves, and took it at huge cost to the native inhabitants. They wanted laborers to work their fields, to build their wealth, and mercilessly spirited away millions of captive Africans to work as slaves, not even seen as human, in their "new" world. It was inevitable, in the sense that asserting domination when we have the means to do so is, it seems, a strong characteristic of our species, at least to date. Even the words juxtaposed together, "slave trade," carry unthinkable suffering and unimaginable cruelty.

And America, North and South, are not alone in this history of usurpation of other peoples' dwelling space and subjugation of others seen as less than human. It goes on to this day. Going back a lot or a little, no civilization is entirely clean in this regard.

Modern civilization, just like in colonial times, needs natural resources to feed its growth. But our consumption dwarfs the scale of colonial times. Civil society needs sources of energy to run its machines, raw materials to feed its factories, and markets in which to sell its goods. It is an organism that needs constant feeding. We now abhor slavery, but we are still uncomfortably close to being enslaved by the mentality of collective rapaciousness and self-righteousness that features our tribe's needs and desires above those we deem less fortunate, less deserving, or less "evolved," whatever form the othering and dehumanizing takes, ignoring once again that them is us.

We suffer from these excesses and atrocities, past and present, that are really travesties of greed and/or ignorance, but that we tend to rationalize as inevitable, as just "human nature." As a country, it feels as if we can no longer afford the karma of such self-centered arrogance, an arrogance that belies our professed ideals of liberty and justice for all, and for life, liberty, and the pursuit of happiness. Wars last days now, or a few weeks, or go on forever. But the war within ourselves and within the human species seems endless.

What is to be done?

Perhaps we need to recognize and purposefully disengage from our past karma and listen carefully inwardly and outwardly for our present and future dharma. Sooner or later, we are going to have to realize, in the sense of make real, the sacred trust our national rhetoric in America extols but so many of our actions belie or betray. For we can no longer afford not to wake up to our truest nature as a species, as a civilization, as a nation of many peoples, and as the only "superpower" of the moment but fading fast. We might do well to recall that the Mongol empire was also the only superpower in its day, as were, to a first approximation, the Egyptians, the Persians, the Greeks, the Romans, the Saracens, the Mayans, and the Incas.

Our opportunity in this era is as a species, not as a superpower.

As a species, we are poised to undergo a quantum leap to another level of being. We are waking up more and more to both the beauty and the good that we bring into the world through our cleverness and our industry and our capacity for love and kindness, and we are also becoming more aware of the need to face up to the harm and suffering we bring into the world through our greed and our heedlessness.

We are at a fecund turning point now, a priceless and delicate juncture between karma and dharma. Karma is the accumulated consequences of past actions in the present moment. Dharma is the conscious embodiment of the inherent radiance of our species, the realization of everything that is intelligent and good and kind and wise in our hearts and minds when we are aligned with the intrinsic lawfulness of the universe. And this includes recognizing our own capacity to generate either heaven or hell, *eudaimonia* or unimaginable suffering in any moment, depending on how mindful or mindless we are, how much we are either free or ensnared by wanting, by craving, by fear, by our own delusions, by our own far-too-small-and-small-minded sense of self. This is the gift of mindfulness when we nurture it in our personal lives and embody it in our relationship with the world. It also includes recognizing and honoring the very real shadow side of our own nature, without succumbing to it.

The challenge is nothing less than a wake-up call to our species. The choice is this: We can seize the opportunity to rotate in consciousness, to undergo a quantum leap through cultivating our capacity for sentience, for mindfulness, for awareness, for compassion, even though it is messy and requires considerable motivation and ongoing effort and practice as individual people, as nations, and as planetary citizens, given all the karma we carry; or we can suffer the consequences, ever more terrifying, of our heedlessness, our ignoring of what is most important, most fundamental for life on Earth at this critical juncture to flourish and for us all to pursue our possibilities to their fullest and their wisest. These alternatives are being played out moment by moment by moment as life unfolds, as they always have. It is just that the stakes keep getting higher and higher as the rate of change itself grows faster and faster, and our technologies provide ever new ways of causing mischief, harm, or unimaginable benefit, often hard to differentiate and disentangle.

We are longing to taste and become intimate with an authentic way to be in this world, and to be true to our deepest nature as human beings. You might even say we are starving for authentic experience, for a deep and embodied authenticity. We are starving for freedom, for deep connection with ourselves and the world and for the liberty to be as we are—with both its inward and its outward promise. To taste liberty, we must liberate ourselves from our own small mindedness and closed hearts, and celebrate that freedom in the community of our own being and in our belonging, in the sangha and sanctuary of each other. Ironically, we yearn for an intrinsic equanimity, connectedness, and actual happiness that have been our birthright all along. True well-being, independent of circumstances, has proven elusive and ephemeral because we have been so lost in our own minds' desires, by virtue of having, to one degree or another, lost our minds, forgotten our hearts, and reified a far-too-small sense of self.

And how do we go about tasting that liberty, that robust well-being? The same way you get to Carnegie Hall. Practice, practice, practice. Mindfulness, mindfulness, mindfulness. And as Rumi put it, by letting the beauty we love (and the beauty we are) be what we do.

The past twelve thousand years of civilization, of growing into ourselves, has been a time of incubation and gestation. Now, a new emergence is not only possible but necessary—a quantum leap for *Homo sapiens sapiens*, a chance to taste what is here to be tasted, to know what is ours to know, in this very generation and the next few to follow. We need intentionality and resolve for this, as well as patience and wisdom. We need to think in terms of several hundred years rather than just the next few. The native peoples of America speak of true stewardship of the earth requiring keeping in mind the well-being of those at least seven generations beyond ours. We would do well to tend the world in such a way. After all, they—those humans yet to come—are us.

# REFLECTIONS ON THE NATURE OF NATURE AND WHERE WE FIT IN

When I was twelve, a small group of boys whose families spent summers in Woods Hole, Massachusetts, because their parents had ties to the laboratories there, used to hang out in what was in those days the coolest place in town, the MBL (Marine Biological Laboratories) Club; that is, when we weren't tooling around on our bikes or at the beach or going home for lunch. In between Ping-Pong games and the like, in rooms decorated with colored glass globes, starfish, and big crab shells hanging suspended beneath the ceiling in fishing nets, in cozy alcoves lined with musty books and built-in cushioned love seats and chess sets scattered about, I remember long conversations about big topics. Jaskin's Drug Store stocked a whole rotating rack of Mentor paperbacks for fifty cents each, with titles such as *One, Two, Three...Infinity* and *The Birth and Death of the Sun* by George Gamow, and *Frontiers of Astronomy* by Fred Hoyle. We bought them up and read them voraciously and were enthralled. We would sit around drinking Cokes from green bottles we got from the big red machine in the basement of the MBL, where you had to pull the large handle around to the right after putting in your nickel to make the bottle drop down, reading out loud to each other and debating the big bang and the steady state theories, the nature of the universe and consciousness, and what it all meant for our lives. I still have my copy of *One, Two, Three...Infinity*. It has that old paperback smell, its pages yellowed and brittle, its spine broken.

Fast-forward (we all know that image, although it would not have made any sense in 1956) to now. In a lovely book that is the modern counterpart to those we used to read as kids, called *The Elegant Universe,* by the theoretical physicist Brian Greene, we are informed that the constraints imposed by superstring theory require the universe to be eleven-dimensional. This may be a little hard for some of us to absorb, given that we have barely come to terms with Einstein's insight that the universe consists of four dimensions, the fourth being time.

Nevertheless, physicists now believe (if this is the right term ever when speaking of physicists) or are giving serious consideration to the possibility that the universe that came into being with the big bang out of "nothing" in one infinitely short, unthinkably brief moment that defined the beginning of time some 13.7 billion years ago (stranger than any ancient creation myth, Babylonian or otherwise), is an eleven-dimensional universe.

Apparently seven of the original eleven dimensions failed to "unfurl" at that moment of creation, giving us the appearance of the three we know now, plus time. How sad for them to have missed their one chance to manifest. But they are nevertheless still "here," curled up in their primordial potentiality inside and within everything (if we can say that), and they have to be for the universe to "work," for protons to be protons and electrons to be electrons, and quarks to be quarks. All this apparently comes out of the math itself, the math of the universe, which is an interesting notion in itself. Our senses, of course, are only geared for three dimensions, or perhaps four, depending on just how sensitive you are.

Fast-forward again from the moment of the big bang to ourselves. Our bodies are whole galaxies of their own on every level, right down to the cellular and sub-cellular. These bodies that we say are "ours" are veritable universes really, made up of unimaginable numbers of atoms, to say nothing of their constituent elementary particles, in a continual dynamic exchange with the rest of the larger universe in which they are nested. And once you are at the atomic level, it turns out that they are actually almost entirely empty space, since the atoms themselves are almost entirely empty space, only tiny condensations of energy fields into what we tend to think of as particles but are equally well described as probability waves, in any event, extremely concentrated loci of huge energies in the nucleus of each atom.

So the big bang, and a lot of time, gave rise to human bodies, and also apparently, although mysteriously, to minds, to sentience. How wonderful. How unfathomable. How unbelievable. It is as if we are the (or one) way for the hydrogen atom—or the quark, or the string, or whatever is most fundamental in this world (the primordial impulse that disgorged the universe out of nothing and nowhere)—to eventually look at itself, and know itself in some way, through what we call consciousness, or sentience. Sentience is a huge question mark for cognitive neuroscience, and no one, as we have already observed (see Book 3, "Sentience"), has the slightest idea how one goes from matter and neurons to the subjective experience of a textured world, from photons of a certain wavelength to the color "blue" as we perceive it experientially, to say nothing of the world which seems to be "out there" but which is only "out there" in relationship to our experiencing of it "in here" (see Book 1, p. xxv). It seems that it is *the relationship* that is most important, not the separation. The separation is in some way illusory, only conventionally tenable and convenient to sometimes speak of. So explaining sentience any time soon may be a long way off, as Yogi Berra might have put it.

What's more, this sentience and its extended sensing capacity, amplified by telescopes, spectrophotometers, and other instruments we send out into space on satellites, or with others here on earth, some deep underground, now seems to be finding that only a very small fraction—astronomers say about 4 percent—of the mass and energy of the universe is in the form of matter as we know it. Almost a quarter of it is what is called "dark matter," and so far, no one really knows what it might consist of, but if it weren't there apparently the galaxies would fall apart. The rest, around 72 percent is "dark energy," which seems to be pushing the universe apart at an increasingly accelerating rate, a sort of anti-gravity. What is more, the notion that there is only one "universe" is currently seen as fairly quaint and unlikely. Serious scientists now speak of a *multiverse* of universes, and have compelling arguments for why this might be a better and more accurate description of whatever we mean by "reality," although by definition, we may not be able to demonstrate the presence of those other universes, at least directly.*

In any event, coming back to us and to our capacity for sensing and knowing, the emergence of the complex—like life and sentience—from the less complex, like inert matter, is one way of looking at the interplay of chaos, complexity, and order in attempting to explain such phenomena to ourselves conceptually, rationally. But because it all seems to "originate" at the moment of the big bang, we are still faced with something coming out of nothing, space coming out of "before space" and time beginning at a certain point, before which there was none, and all matter coming out of nowhere as infinite pure energy. Hmmmm. Why isn't all this turning on troves of kids to a love of science? I would think it would.

Another way to look at things says that something cannot come out of nothing, and especially that consciousness cannot come out of matter. That is more of a Buddhist view.

It is fascinating to have these two vital ways of exploring the nature of reality and the nature of mind in dynamic dialogue, as they are in this era, thanks in large measure to the Dalai Lama's lifelong interest in science and how things work.†

---

* See Tegmark, M. *Our Mathematical Universe: My Quest for the Ultimate Nature of Reality*, Knopf, New York, 2014; Greene, B. *The Hidden Reality: Parallel Universes and the Deep Laws of the Cosmos*, Knopf, New York, 2011.; and Randall, L. *Knocking on Heaven's Door: How Physics and Scientific Thinking Illuminated the Universe*, HarperCollins, New York, 2011.

† See the books put out by the Mind and Life Institute (www.mindandlife.org) on these various conversations between the Dalai Lama and Buddhist monks and nuns and scholars, and scientists from various disciplines, mostly cognitive neuroscience, psychology, biology, physics, and philosophy. See for example, Hasenkamp, W. (ed.). *The Monastery*

*There was something formless and perfect*
*before the universe was born.*
*It is serene. Empty.*
*Solitary. Unchanging.*
*Infinite. Eternally present.*
*It is the mother of the universe.*
*For lack of a better name,*
*I call it the Tao.*

LAO TZU, *Tao Te Ching*


Consider one last time the "universe" that is us. On one level, our body is almost entirely empty space (or fields) with rare foci of highly condensed energy, which we call mass. Going up in scale, these foci are first strings (if string theory in one form or another is even remotely correct, which at the moment is far from certain), then quarks, electrons, protons, and neutrons, then atoms. Then, going up still further, we notice associations of atoms into small molecules, and mid-size molecules, macro-molecules (such as enzymes and proteins), and mega-molecules such as DNA, the mother lode of "software," so to speak, driving and regulating the life-universe on this planet. Then there are mega-associations of molecules (organelles) such as ribosomes and endoplasmic reticulum and Golgi apparati (don't the very words sound mysterious and mellifluous?).

All this describes some small fraction of the contents of one cell in a body that, as we have seen, is made up of unimaginable numbers (between ten and one hundred trillion) of cells, all originating from one cell, the fertilized egg that itself came from two cells, one from

---

*and the Microscope: Conversations with the Dalai Lama on Mind, Mindfulness, and the Nature of Reality*, Yale University Press, New Haven, CT, 2017; and Harrington, A. and Zajonc, A. (eds.). *The Dalai Lama at MIT*, Harvard University Press, Cambridge, MA, 2008; https://www.mindandlife.org/books/.

each parent universe, that came together because our parents' bodies, in the standard version, came together.*

Do we ever *experience* this, know ourselves in this way, even for a moment? And I don't mean solely through thought—although deep thought and some knowledge of the physics and chemistry and biology and cognitive science can help—but through awareness, through feeling and sensing, through being embodied and inviting our minds to inhabit and fill the body, from the envelope of the skin right down to the muscles and joints and bones and liver and lungs, and sometimes throbbing genitals, always throbbing heart and blood and brain, and everything else we might want to invoke in terms of emotions, organs, and tissues, right down to the cells themselves, right down still further to the chromosomes and ribosomes and enzymes busily working away (if we can call it working) in this on-this-level-mostly-water world, right down to the molecules, atoms, quarks, and strings and the emptiness between them and within them, including the seven not unfurled (how else to speak of them, un-unfurled?) dimensions of reality or nature itself.

In other words, can we realize all that we are, at the level of the material and the non-material, object and subject, and beyond subject and object, in this very moment, simultaneously? Can we see, realize, attain, absorb the living miracle and mystery of it, that it all works, that we can think, that we can move, and walk, and talk, digest our food, make love, have babies and nurture them to adulthood, find food and meaning, make art and music, find each other, take care of each other, work together, and ultimately perhaps, even know ourselves?

And can we also realize, in the nick of time perhaps, given the urgency and the high stakes for humanity, that, in many ways, we are ironically but unwittingly poisoning ourselves and the biosphere,

---

* And that is not counting the microbiome, bacteria on or within the body that equal or outnumber, according to various estimates, our own human cells. See, for example: https://www.ncbi.nlm.nih.gov/pmc/articles/PMC4991899/.

both psychically and materially, out of our endless and magnificent but unexamined precocity, out of our fear and our greediness, and the cleverness of our minds and our industriousness, a cleverness that turns dangerous when we become attached, entrenched, absorbed, delighted with parts but uninterested in wholes and larger wholes?

In the past, humanity didn't know much about how our activity affects the planet as a whole, and the nature of the dis-ease and disease it is currently suffering from. Now at least we debate the health status of the world and monitor aspects of its vital signs, and ponder their meaning and potential consequences. We can now be mindful of the planet and its health, and of our effects on its well-being. All in all, perhaps that attention and our caring are in themselves signs of intelligent life on this planet—hopefully coming into its own as embodied wisdom and, inseparably, as compassion for all life, for all sentience. That includes our own, and our children's.

# Hidden Dimensions Unfurled

It strikes me that the metaphor of hidden dimensions that have somehow not "unfurled" has practical applications in our lives. If physicists can think seriously in such strange ways, perhaps we all might as well, and thereby take a closer look at what is right beneath our noses.

For we might say that there are multiple dimensions in our own lives that are tightly curled up within us and for whatever reasons have not had the opportunity to unfurl, at least so far. If they did, perhaps it would come as quite a big bang in our own lives. Many stories speak of revelation and clarity in the meditative traditions in just that way, as sudden "explosions" of insight. They are hardly stranger than what science has been cooking up for us.

One such hidden dimension would be the present moment. The present moment is always right here, yet more often than not it is not apparent to us and therefore, practically speaking, unavailable—that is, we cannot avail ourselves of it. Its rich dimensionality is hidden and unknown in the press of our preoccupations with getting somewhere else, to a better moment or an end-result, speeding through the present without noticing it or that we are always in it, there being literally no place else to go or to be, no other time to occupy—unless we lose our minds and forget our hearts.

Might this dimension that is the present moment unfurl for us? It might. It might.

What would it take? How about stopping, looking, and listening? How about coming to our senses?

Earlier on (see Book 2, "Being Seen" and Book 3, "Attaining Place"), we dropped in on T. S. Eliot's sumptuous banquet in the *Four Quartets* and helped ourselves to the dessert. Still, it may take some time, if we have the stomach for it, to digest those immortal lines:

*Not known because not looked for,*
*But heard, half-heard in the stillness*
*Between two waves of the sea.*
*Quick, now, here, now always,*
*A condition of complete simplicity*
*(Costing not less than everything)*

The power and profundity of our own embodied wakefulness embedded within the present moment is inconceivable, just as inconceivable for us as the huge energy of the vacuum or the tininess of un-unfurled dimensions deep inside our atoms or nested within the fabric of space itself. In the case of the present moment, there is no way to believe in it, and no need to. One need only experience it and see for oneself how it might add back a dimension to living that accords us other degrees of freedom as well, whole new realms and ways to inhabit our lives and our world for the brief moments we are here that sum so quickly to what we call a lifetime and that are so easily missed. That is a banquet we are all called to, a repast where, moment by moment, you are invited, as Derek Walcott so beautifully put it, to: "Sit. Feast on your life."

Picture an incomprehensible vastness of space, with no beginning, no end, and no center. Vast emptiness, and yet full of discrete foci of matter, galaxies with unimaginable numbers of stars, these galaxies themselves clustered over unthinkable distances and times in what look like bubbles, membranes drawn over emptiness, yet also receding from each other at incredible speeds in an accelerating expansion that can be extrapolated backward 13.7 billion years, at which point, as we have seen, all matter and energy, space and time must have been condensed into a droplet of no dimension whatsoever and nothing outside of it because there is no outside to the universe.

Picture in this incomprehensible vastness of space and unimaginable timelessness of time the Earth, serendipitously slotted at a cozy distance from a relatively young and unremarkable star at the edge of one such galaxy, in what is sometimes referred to as the Goldilocks sweet spot (not too hot and not too cold for the emergence of complex life forms), said planet itself formed approximately 4 billion years ago along with the sun and the other planets in our solar system out of thin clouds of atoms heavier than hydrogen and helium that could only have been formed in the furnaces of earlier generations of stars and in the spectacular explosions of some of them as they burned up their hydrogen and ultimately capitulated to the unrelenting attractive force of their own massiveness, namely what we call gravity. Picture unimaginable stretches of time on the early Earth with landscapes inhabited by no creatures, tectonic plates forming and rearranging themselves over eons, the whole slowly incubating life—life in the sea, life on the land, life in the air—at first extraordinarily simple life forms and later, more and more complex forms, and in what has been, by comparison, only a few incomprehensibly short seconds, giving rise to ourselves, to human life as we know it. Even if we date the origins of humanity back three hundred thousand years or so, which is the best guesstimate at the moment for our species, it is still less than an eye blink in the vastness of time.

Marvel for a moment at the flowering of life on this sphere of blue and green and white and brown, hanging in the vast emptiness, the boundlessness, the blackness of space. And marvel for a moment at the fact that, in a dwelling near the coast of an enormous continent of tortured rock floating on a core of more of the same in a molten condition, and beneath that, a core of molten iron, these sentences can be written on a machine that receives the pressure of fingers, in conjunction with eyes that can see the human-made flat screen where the words unfold in pixels, words that clothe currents of organized energy we call thoughts and feelings, which magically emerge from a mind which itself has no clue how this is happening. All this is dependent in some mysterious way on a three-pound organ contained within the cranium, the human brain—an organ with an astonishing level of complexity and interconnectedness made out of living tissues and executing synaptic transmissions, modulations, inhibitions, veritably the most highly complex organization of matter in the known universe. And all this evolved out of small tree-dwelling primates in Africa a long long time ago, by our paltry standards of time.

Let's reflect on that inheritance one more time: we are talking about the most complex arrangement of matter and energy flow in the known-by-us universe, residing right here underneath our very own cranium and extending itself throughout these miraculous heads and bodies of ours.

And yet, we can go through the day more or less on autopilot, worrying endlessly: about money and whether we can pay the bills, about our children and how they will fare in this world, about whether or not we are happy or will ever be happy, about whether people like us or not, whether we are as successful as we should be, whether we will ever get the love and acceptance we long for, or whether we will have any time for ourselves in the press of everything on our endless to-do lists and given the amount of time we spend gazing at screens. We worry about the economy. We worry about our bodies and our minds, about the future and even the past (in the sense that we gnaw on it like a dog worries a bone). We worry about illness, about aging, about losing our senses as we perceive our eyesight, or our hearing, or our ability to sense the ground through our feet in decline. We worry about having no time, about needing more time, about having too much time, about wishing things were different, somehow better, somehow more satisfying. And sooner or later, we get around to worrying about death.

We also worry about this world we live in, which sometimes seems so cruel and senseless, our leaders at times unimaginably mindless and grotesquely and dangerously unwedded to facts, where countless people live in poverty and squalor, often with no political voice until, like magic, they sometimes find it for themselves. We worry about this world where suspicion, violence, and aggression are all too commonly perpetrated on others, on ourselves at times, and on the natural world that we continue to despoil as a by-product of our natural drive to make things and to sell them, ratcheted up by ambition to corner some market, enhance some returns, carve out some niche, beat out our competitors, make America great again while we are at it, acquire more money and more stuff, and hopefully, as a result of all that, to find happiness.

Haven't we lost perspective just a tad? Are we not ignoring or forgetting to see and to feel the whole of our condition as individuals and as a species? Are we not also ignoring our smallness, our insignificance, our utter temporariness? Or are we perhaps trying to compensate unconsciously for our vulnerabilities and insecurities by insisting on controlling and dominating nature instead of remembering that we are born of and are seamlessly interwoven into it, and so the most important thing might be to know ourselves and something of our own nature before we act out of unexamined motives—and before we run out of time?

Are we not also ignoring our beauty and our remarkable potential, a mysterious flowering of possibility for true intelligence in this more-than-strange universe that is our home and that we might learn to be more at home in? Are we not ignoring the miracle of the human form, this thimbleful of atoms birthed in stars that is the human body, the utter gift of a human life and the possibility of its being lived fully and well, in touch with rather than ignoring our fundamental creativity and the mystery of our sentience, our consciousness, our presence here, our absolute need for each other, our ability to look in awe and wonder and in knowing upon the universe within which we emerged and which we now inhabit?

From the point of view of the universe, from the perspective of infinite space and unimaginable time, what happens on this small planet is of no consequence. But it is of major consequence to us since we are here, if briefly, and will be passing whatever we do with the world and learn from it on to future generations. Might it not be time for us to capture the full spectrum of our inherent capabilities, to explore and grow into the fullness of what it might mean to be human while we still have the chance?

There is considerable evidence that we are approaching an inflection point in our evolution as a species in the next few decades and centuries, a tipping point. Our precocity as maker and thinker has brought us to the point where we can influence our own genes, pursue genetically extended longevity if not immortality, experiment with silicon/living biology interfaces for information storage and retrieval (who would turn down the opportunity of a memory upgrade if such were possible?), design machines that may soon "think" better and faster than we do, and maybe someday will feel as well, or at least simulate it increasingly convincingly, and maybe, in the not-too-distant future, make programmable and self-replicating machines and robots so small that we can swallow them and have them literally keep the body in shape, molecule by molecule, perhaps "forever."

In the face of such eventualities, and the many others that are so far inconceivable but bound to emerge rapidly in this culture where whatever we can conceive of doing that is technologically possible sooner or later seems to get done, even if few ever get to voice a say in the matter, and only a few think it a good idea. The prophets of the Old Testament railed at the heedlessness of their own people. Were they alive today, they might rail with equal vim and vigor at our heedlessness as a species now. Whether there are voices that can be heard above the mindless din or not, humanity itself can now no longer afford our own massive interior ignoring of who we are and where we live, nor the ignoring of the consequences of our individual and collective actions, given where our precocity has taken us since those ancient, biblical times that were only a short while ago.

Perhaps it is time for us to own and fully inhabit the name we have given ourselves as a species (*Homo sapiens sapiens*—the species that knows and knows that it knows, in other words, which is characterized by the capacity for awareness and meta-awareness*). This inevitably invites us to own our sentience, and come to our senses, literally and metaphorically, while there is still time for us to do so. And while we might not realize it, that time, by all reckoning, is shorter than we think. And the stakes higher. What is at stake, finally, is none other than our hearts, our very humanity, our species, and our world. What is available to us is the full spectrum of who and what we are. What is required is nothing special, simply that, as human beings, we start paying attention more systematically, wake up to things as they are,

---

* Not cognition and meta-cognition, since our knowing is far more multidimensional than mere cognition, wonderful as our capacity for thinking is. As we have seen, *sapiens* also means knowing through tasting, as we have seen, a placeholder for all our senses, far more in number than the conventional five.

and act with integrity, with wisdom, with care and caring. Befriending your mind and your life and world through the daily cultivation of mindfulness as a love affair with the present moment, with life itself, and with the domain of ongoing learning and growing, healing and transformation, is very likely an essential element in cultivating that embodied wakefulness and wisdom. If we take care of that, and are willing to fully inhabit this moment, all else will follow.

# ACKNOWLEDGMENTS

Since the origins of these four volumes go back a long way, there are a number of people to whom I wish to express my gratitude and indebtedness for their many contributions at various stages of the writing and publishing of these books.

For the initial volume, published in 2005, I would like to thank my dharma brother, Larry Rosenberg of the Cambridge Insight Meditation Center, as well as Larry Horwitz, and my father-in-law, the late Howard Zinn, for reading the entire manuscript back in the day and sharing their keen and creative insights with me. My thanks as well to Alan Wallace, Arthur Zajonc, Doug Tanner, and Richard Davidson and to Will Kabat-Zinn and Myla Kabat-Zinn for reading portions of the manuscript and giving me their wise council and feedback. I also thank the original publisher, Bob Miller, and the original editor, Will Schwalbe, now both at Flatiron Books, for their support and friendship, then and now.

Deep and special appreciation, gratitude, and indebtedness to my editor of the first volume, Michelle Howry, executive editor at Hachette Books, who helped midwife the form of the entire series; to Lauren Hummel for her key contributions to making sure all went well, and skillfully keeping all of the moving parts of this project on track; and to the entire Hachette team that worked so cooperatively and effectively on this series. Also, deep appreciation to Mauro DiPreta, vice president and publisher of Hachette Books, who stepped in to shepherd the last three volumes through the publication process when Michelle moved on.

While I have received support, encouragement, and advice from many, of course any inaccuracies or shortcomings in the text are entirely my own.

I wish to express enduring gratitude and respect to all my teaching colleagues, past and present, in the Stress Reduction Clinic and the Center for Mindfulness and, more recently, also to those teachers and researchers who are part of the CFM's global network of affiliate institutions. All have literally and metaphorically dedicated their lives and their passion to this work. At the time of the original book, those who had taught MBSR in the Stress Reduction Clinic for varying periods of time from 1979 to 2005 were Saki Santorelli, Melissa Blacker, Florence Meleo-Meyer, Elana Rosenbaum, Ferris Buck Urbanowski, Pamela Erdmann, Fernando de Torrijos, James Carmody, Danielle Levi Alvares, George Mumford, Diana Kamila, Peggy Roggenbuck-Gillespie, Debbie Beck, Zayda Vallejo, Barbara Stone, Trudy Goodman, Meg Chang, Larry Rosenberg, Kasey Carmichael, Franz Moekel, the late Ulli Kesper-Grossman, Maddy Klein, Ann Soulet, Joseph Koppel, the late Karen Ryder, Anna Klegon, Larry Pelz, Adi Bemak, Paul Galvin, and David Spound.

From 2005 to 2017, my admiration and gratitude go to the teachers at the Center for Mindfulness and its affiliate programs: Florence Meleo-Meyers, Lynn Koerbel, Elana Rosenbaum, Carolyn West, Bob Stahl, Meg Chang, Zayda Vallejo, Brenda Fingold, Dianne Horgan, Judson Brewer, Margaret Fletcher, Patti Holland, Rebecca Eldridge, Ted Meissner, Anne Twohig, Ana Arrabe, Beth Mulligan, Bonita Jones, Carola Garcia, Gustavo Diex, Beatriz Rodriguez, Melissa Tefft, Janet Solyntjes, Rob Smith, Jacob Piet, Claude Maskens, Charlotte Borch-Jacobsen, Christiane Wolf, Kate Mitcheom, Bob Linscott, Laurence Magro, Jim Colosi, Julie Nason, Lone Overby Fjorback, Dawn MacDonald, Leslie Smith Frank, Ruth Folchman, Colleen Camenisch, Robin Boudette, Eowyn Ahlstrom, Erin Woo, Franco Cuccio, Geneviève Hamelet, Gwenola Herbette, and Ruth Whitall. Florence Meleo-Meyer and Lynn Koerbel were outstanding leaders and nurturers of the global network of MBSR teachers at the CFM.

Profound appreciation to all those who contributed so critically in so many different ways to the administration of the MBSR Clinic and the Center for Mindfulness in Medicine, Health Care, and Society and to their various research and clinical endeavors from the very beginning: Norma Rosiello, Kathy Brady, Brian Tucker, Anne Skillings, Tim Light, Jean Baril, Leslie Lynch, Carol Lewis, Leigh Emery, Rafaela Morales, Roberta Lewis, Jen Gigliotti, Sylvia Ciario, Betty Flodin, Diane Spinney, Carol Hester, Carol Mento, Olivia Hobletzell, the late Narina Hendry, Marlene Samuelson, Janet Parks, Michael Bratt, Marc Cohen, and Ellen Wingard. For the period up to the spring of 2018, I extend my gratitude to Judson Brewer, Dianne Horgan, Florence Meleo-Meyer, Lynn Koerbel, Jean Baril, Jacqueline Clark, Tony Maciag, Ted Meissner, Jessica Novia, Maureen Titus, Beverly Walton, Ashley Gladden, Lynne Littizzio, Nicole Rocijewicz, and Jean Welker.

On the research side, robust appreciation for the contributions of the members of Judson Brewer's lab: Remko van Lutterveld, Prasanta Pal, Michael Datko, Andrea Ruf, Susan Druker, Ariel Beccia, Alexandra Roy, Hanif Benoit, Danny Theisen, and Carolyn Neal.

In the spring of 2018, the Center for Mindfulness underwent what I like to think of as a process of binary fission, with a number of people migrating to Brown University to establish a parallel and complementary mindfulness center and research program there under the aegis of the School of Public Health and the Medical School. I wish to express my gratitude to all involved in both institutions for what has been and what is yet to come in terms of clinical and professional training programs, research directions, and collaborative possibilities.

Finally, I would also like to express my gratitude and respect for the thousands of people everywhere around the world who work in or are researching mindfulness-based approaches in medicine, psychiatry, psychology, health care, education, the law, social justice, refugee healing in the face of trauma and sometimes genocide (as in South Sudan), childbirth and parenting, the workplace, government, prisons, and other facets of society, and who take care to honor the dharma in its universal depth and beauty in doing so. You know who you are, whether you are named here or not! And if you are not, it is only due to my own shortcomings and the limits of space. I want to explicitly honor the work of Paula Andrea Ramirez Diazgranados in Columbia and South Sudan; Hui Qi Tong in the U.S. and China; Kevin Fong, Roy Te Chung Chen, Tzungkuen Wen, Helen Ma, Jin Mei Hu, and Shih Shih Ming in China, Taiwan, and Hong Kong; Heyoung Ahn in Korea; Junko Bickel and Teruro Shiina in Japan; Leena Pennenen in Finland; Simon Whitesman and Linda Kantor in South Africa; Claude Maskens, Gwénola Herbette, Edel Max, Caroline Lesire, and Ilios Kotsou in Belgium; Jean-Gérard Bloch, Geneviève Hamelet, Marie-Ange Pratili, and Charlotte Borch-Jacobsen in France; Katherine Bonus, Trish Magyari, Erica Sibinga, David Kearney, Kurt Hoelting, Carolyn McManus, Mike Brumage, Maureen Strafford, Amy Gross, Rhonda Magee, George Mumford, Carl Fulwiler, Maria Kluge, Mick Krasner, Trish Luck, Bernice Todres, Ron Epstein, and Representative Tim Ryan in the U.S.: Paul Grossman, Maria Kluge, Sylvia Wiesman-Fiscalini, Linda Hehrhaupt, and Petra Meibert in Germany; Joke Hellemans, Johan Tinge, and Anna Speckens in Holland; Beatrice Heller and Regula Saner in Switzerland; Rebecca Crane, Willem Kuyken, John Teasdale, Mark Williams, Chris Cullen, Richard Burnett, Jamie Bristow, Trish Bartley, Stewart Mercer, Chris Ruane, Richard Layard, Guiaume Hung, and Ahn Nguyen in the UK; Zindel Segal and Norm Farb in Canada; Gabor Fasekas in Hungary; Macchi dela Vega, Clara Badino, and Marina Lisenberg in Argentina; Johan Bergstad, Anita Olsson, Angeli Holmstedt; Ola Schenström, and Camilla Sköld in Sweden; Andries Kroese in Norway; Jakob Piet and Lone Overby Fjorback in Denmark; and Franco Cuccio in Italy. May your work continue to reach those who are most in need of it, touching, clarifying, and nurturing what is deepest and best in us all, and thus contributing, in ways little and big to the healing and transformation that humanity so sorely longs for and aspires to.

## The Roots of Mindfulness Meditation

Amero, B. *Small Boat, Great Mountain: Theravadan Reflections on the Great Natural Perfection*, Abhayagiri Monastic Foundation, Redwood Valley, CA, 2003.

Analayo, B. *Early Buddhist Meditation Studies*, Barre Center for Buddhist Studies, Barre, MA, 2017.

Analayo, B. *Mindfully Facing Disease and Death: Compassionate Advice from Early Buddhist Texts*, Windhorse, Cambridge, UK, 2016.

Analayo, B. *Mindfulness of Breathing: A Practice Guide and Translations*, Windhorse, Cambridge, UK, 2019.

Analayo, B. *Satipatthana: The Direct Path to Realization*, Windhorse, Cambridge, UK, 2008.

Analayo, B. *Satipatthana Meditation: A Practice Guide*, Windhorse, Cambridge, UK, 2018.

Armstrong, G. *Emptiness: A Practical Guide for Meditators I*, Wisdom, Somerville, MA, 2017.

Beck, C. *Nothing Special: Living Zen*, HarperCollins, San Francisco, 1993.

Buswell, R. B., Jr. *Tracing Back the Radiance: Chinul's Korean Way of Zen*, Kuroda Institute, U of Hawaii Press, Honolulu, 1991.

Goldstein, J. *Mindfulness: A Practical Guide to Awakening*, Sounds True, Boulder, CO, 2013.

Goldstein, J. *One Dharma: The Emerging Western Buddhism*, HarperCollins, San Francisco, 2002.

Goldstein, J. and Kornfield, J. *Seeking the Heart of Wisdom: The Path of Insight Meditation*, Shambhala, Boston, 1987.

Gunaratana, H. *Mindfulness in Plain English*, Wisdom, Boston, 1996.

Hanh, T. N. *The Heart of the Buddha's Teachings*, Broadway, New York, 1998.

Hanh, T. N. *How to Love*, Parallax Press, Berkeley, 2015

Hanh, T. N. *How to Sit*, Parallax Press, Berkeley, 2014.

Hanh, T. N. *The Miracle of Mindfulness*, Beacon, Boston, 1976.

Kapleau, P. *The Three Pillars of Zen: Teaching, Practice, and Enlightenment*, Random House, New York, 1965, 2000.

Krishnamurti, J. *This Light in Oneself: True Meditation*, Shambhala, Boston, 1999.

Levine, S. *A Gradual Awakening*, Anchor/Doubleday, Garden City, NY, 1979.

Ricard, R. *Happiness*. Little Brown, New York, 2007.

Ricard, R. *Why Meditate?*, Hay House, New York, 2010.

Rinpoche, M. *The Joy of Wisdom*, Harmony Books, New York, 2010.

Rosenberg, L. *Breath by Breath: The Liberating Practice of Insight Meditation*, Shambhala, Boston, 1998.

Rosenberg, L. *Living in the Light of Death: On the Art of Being Truly Alive*, Shambhala, Boston, 2000.

Rosenberg, L. *Three Steps to Awakening: A Practice for Bringing Mindfulness to Life*, Shambhala, Boston, 2013.

Salzberg, S. *Lovingkindness*, Shambhala, Boston, 1995.

Salzberg, S. *Real Love: The Art of Mindful Connection*, Flatiron Books, New York, 2017.

Sheng-yen, C. *Hoofprints of the Ox: Principles of the Chan Buddhist Path*, Oxford University Press, New York, 2001.

Soeng, M. *The Heart of the Universe: Exploring the Heart Sutra*. Wisdom, Somerville, MA, 2010.

Soeng, M. *Trust in Mind: The Rebellion of Chinese Zen*. Wisdom, Somerville, MA, 2004.

Sumedo, A. *The Mind and the Way: Buddhist Reflections on Life*, Wisdom, Boston, 1995.

Suzuki, S. *Zen Mind, Beginner's Mind*, Weatherhill, New York, 1970.

Thera, N. *The Heart of Buddhist Meditation: The Buddha's Way of Mindfulness*, Red Wheel/Weiser, San Francisco, 1962, 2014.

Tulku Urgyen. *Rainbow Painting*, Rangjung Yeshe, Boudhanath, Nepal, 1995.

## MBSR

Brandsma, R. *The Mindfulness Teaching Guide: Essential Skills and Competencies for Teaching Mindfulness-Based Interventions*, New Harbinger, Oakland, CA, 2017.

Kabat-Zinn, J. *Full Catastrophe Living: Using the Wisdom of Your Body and Mind to Face Stress, Pain, and Illness*, revised and updated edition, Random House, New York, 2013.

Lehrhaupt, L. and Meibert, P. *Mindfulness-Based Stress Reduction: The MBSR Program for Enhancing Health and Vitality*, New World Library, Novato, CA, 2017.

Mulligan, B. A. *The Dharma of Modern Mindfulness: Discovering the Buddhist Teachings at the Heart of Mindfulness-Based Stress Reduction*, New Harbinger, Oakland, CA, 2017.

Rosenbaum, E. *The Heart of Mindfulness-Based Stress Reduction: An MBSR Guide for Clinicians and Clients*, Pesi Publishing, Eau Claire, WI, 2017.

Stahl, B. and Goldstein, E. *A Mindfulness-Based Stress Reduction Workbook*, New Harbinger, Oakland, CA, 2010.

Stahl, B., Meleo-Meyer, F., and Koerbel, L. *A Mindfulness-Based Stress Reduction Workbook for Anxiety*, New Harbinger, Oakland, CA, 2014.

## Other Applications of Mindfulness

Baer, R. A. (ed.). *Mindfulness-Based Treatment Approaches: Clinician's Guide to Evidence Base and Applications*, Academic Press, Waltham, MA, 2014.

Bardacke, N. *Mindfulness Birthing: Training the Mind, Body, and Heart for Childbirth and Beyond*, HarperCollins, New York, 2012.

Bartley, T. *Mindfulness: A Kindly Approach to Cancer*, Wiley-Blackwell, West Sussex, UK, 2016.

Bartley, T. *Mindfulness-Based Cognitive Therapy for Cancer*, Wiley-Blackwell, West Sussex, UK, 2012.

Bays, J. C. *Mindful Eating: A Guide to Rediscovering a Healthy and Joyful Relationship with Food*, Shambhala, Boston, 2009, 2017.

Bays, J. C. *Mindfulness on the Go: Simple Meditation Practices You Can Do Anywhere*, Shambhala, Boston, 2014.

Biegel, G. *The Stress-Reduction Workbook for Teens: Mindfulness Skills to Help You Deal with Stress*, New Harbinger, Oakland, CA, 2017.

Bögels, S. and Restifo, K. *Mindful Parenting: A Guide for Mental Health Practitioners*, Springer, New York, 2014.

Brantley, J. *Calming Your Anxious Mind: How Mindfulness and Compassion Can Free You from Anxiety, Fear, and Panic*, New Harbinger, Oakland, CA, 2003.

Brewer, Judson. *The Craving Mind: From Cigarettes to Smartphones to Love—Why We Get Hooked and How We Can Break Bad Habits*, Yale University Press, New Haven, 2017.

Brown, K. W., Creswell, J. D., and Ryan, R. M. (eds). *Handbook of Mindfulness: Theory, Research, and Practice*, Guilford, New York, 2015.

Carlson, L. and Speca, M. *Mindfulness-Based Cancer Recovery: A Step-by-Step MBSR Approach to Help You Cope with Treatment and Reclaim Your Life*, New Harbinger, Oakland, CA, 2010.

Chaskalson, M. *The Mindful Workplace: Developing Resilient Individuals and Resonant Organizations with MBSR*, Wiley-Blackwell, Chichester, UK, 2011.

Crane, R. *Mindfulness-Based Cognitive Therapy*, Routledge, New York, 2017.

Cullen, M. and Pons, G. B. *The Mindfulness-Based Emotional Balance Workbook: An Eight-Week Program for Improved Emotion Regulation and Resilience*, New Harbinger, Oakland, CA, 2015.

del Marmol, G. *No Time to Waste: The Rise of a Regenerative Economy*, Ker Éditions, Hévillers, Belgium, 2017

Epstein, M. *Thoughts Without a Thinker,* Basic Books, New York, 1995.

Epstein, R. *Attending: Medicine, Mindfulness, and Humanity,* Scribner, New York, 2017.

Ergas, O. *Reconstructing "Education" Through Mindful Attention: Positioning the Mind at the Center of Curriculum and Pedagogy,* Palgrave Macmillan, London, UK, 2017.

Folder, S. *What's Beyond Mindfulness: Waking Up to This Precious Life,* Watkins, London, 2019.

Gazzaley, A. and Rosen, L. D. *The Distracted Mind: Ancient Brains in a High-Tech World,* MIT Press, Cambridge, MA, 2016.

Gelles, D. *Mindful Work: How Meditation Is Changing Business from the Inside Out,* Houghton Mifflin Harcourt, New York, 2015.

Germer, C. *The Mindful Path to Self-Compassion,* Guilford, New York, 2009.

Germer, C. K. and Siegel, R. D. (eds.). *Wisdom and Compassion in Psychotherapy: Deepening Mindfulness in Clinical Practice,* Guilford, New York, 2012.

Germer, C. K., Siegel, R. D., and Fulton, P. R. (eds.). *Mindfulness and Psychotherapy,* Guilford, New York, 2005

Goleman, D. *Destructive Emotions: How We Can Heal Them,* Bantam, New York, 2003.

Goleman, G, and Davidson, R. J. *Altered Traits: Science Reveals How Meditation Changes Your Mind, Brain, and Body,* Avery/Random House, New York, 2017.

Gunaratana, B. H. *Mindfulness in Plain English,* Wisdom, Somerville, MA, 2002.

Harris, N. B. *The Deepest Well: Healing the Long-term Effects of Childhood Adversity,* Houghton Mifflin Harcourt, Boston, 2018.

Hasenkamp, W. *The Monastery and the Microscope: Conversations with the Dalai Lama on Mind, Mindfulness, and the Nature of Reality,* Yale, New Haven, 2017.

Himmelstein, S. and Saul, S. *Mindfulness-Based Substance Abuse Treatment for Adolescents—A 12 Session Curriculum,* Routledge, New York, 2016.

Jennings, P. *Mindfulness for Teachers: Simple Skills for Peace and Productivity in the Classroom,* W.W. Norton, New York, 2015.

Jones, A. *Beyond Vision: Going Blind, Inner Seeing, and the Nature of the Self,* McGill-Queen's University Press, Montreal, 2018.

Kabat-Zinn, J. *Mindfulness for Beginners: Reclaiming the Present Moment—and Your Life,* Sounds True, Boulder, CO, 2012.

Kabat-Zinn, J. *Wherever You Go, There You Are: Mindfulness Meditation in Everyday Life,* Hachette, 1994, 2005.

Kabat-Zinn, J. and Davidson, R. J. *The Mind's Own Physician: A Scientific Dialogue with the Dalai Lama on the Healing Power of Meditation,* New Harbinger, Oakland, CA, 2011.

Kabat-Zinn, M. and Kabat-Zinn, J. *Everyday Blessings: The Inner Work of Mindful Parenting,* Hachette, New York, 1997, revised 2014.

Kaiser-Greenland, S. *The Mindful Child*, Free Press, New York, 2010.

Kaiser-Greenland, S. *Mindful Games: Sharing Mindfulness and Games with Children, Teen, and Families*, Shambhala, Boulder, CO, 2016.

Kaufman, K. A., Glass, C. R., and Pineau, T. R. *Mindful Sport Performance Enhancement: Mental Training for Athletes and Coaches*, American Psychological Association (APA), Washington, DC, 2018.

King, R. *Mindful of Race: Transforming Racism from the Inside Out*, Sounds True, Boulder, CO, 2018.

Koole, W. *Mindful Leadership: Effective Tools to Help You Focus and Succeed*, Warden Press, Amsterdam, Netherlands, 2014.

Martins, C. *Mindfulness-Based Interventions for Older Adults: Evidence for Practice*, Jessica Kingsley, Philadelphia, PA, 2014.

Marturano, J. *Finding the Space to Lead: A Practical Guide to Mindful Leadership*, Bloomsbury Press, New York, 2014.

Mason-John, V. and Groves, P. *Eight-Step Recovery: Using the Buddha's Teachings to Overcome Addiction*, Windhorse, Cambridge, UK, 2018.

Maul, F. *Radical Responsibility: A Mindfulness-Based Emotional Intelligence Guide for Personal Evolution, Self-Actualization, and Social Transformation*, Sounds True, Boulder, CO, 2019.

McBee, L. *Mindfulness-Based Elder Care: A CAM Model for Frail Elders and Their Caregivers*, Springer, New York, 2008.

McCown, D., Reibel, D., and Micozzi, M. S. (eds.). *Resources for Teaching Mindfulness: An International Handbook*, Springer, New York, 2016.

McCown, D., Reibel, D., and Micozzi, M. S. (eds.). *Teaching Mindfulness: A Practical Guide for Clinicians and Educators*, Springer, New York, 2010.

McManus, C. A. *Group Wellness Programs for Chronic Pain and Disease Management*, Butterworth-Heinemann, St. Louis, MO, 2003.

Miller, L. D. *Effortless Mindfulness: Genuine Mental Health Through Awakened Presence*, Routledge, New York, 2014.

Mumford, G. *The Mindful Athlete: Secrets to Pure Performance*, Parallax Press, Berkeley, 2015.

Penman, D. *The Art of Breathing*, Conari, Newburyport, MA, 2018.

Pollak, S. M., Pedulla, T., and Siegel, R. D. *Sitting Together: Essential Skills for Mindfulness-Based Psychotherapy*, Guilford, New York, 2014.

Rechtschaffen, D. *The Mindful Education Workbook: Lessons for Teaching Mindfulness to Students*, W.W. Norton, New York, 2016.

Rechtschaffen, D. *The Way of Mindful Education: Cultivating Wellbeing in Teachers and Students*, W.W. Norton, New York, 2014.

Rosenbaum, E. *Being Well (Even When You Are Sick): Mindfulness Practices for People with Cancer and Other Serious Illnesses*, Shambala, Boston, 2012.

Rosenbaum, E. *Here for Now: Living Well with Cancer Through Mindfulness*, Satya House, Hardwick, MA, 2005.

Rossy, L. *The Mindfulness-Based Eating Solution: Proven Strategies to End Over-eating, Satisfy Your Hunger, and Savor Your Life*, New Harbinger, Oakland, CA, 2016.

Segal, Z. V., Williams, J.M.G., and Teasdale, J. D. *Mindfulness-Based Cognitive Therapy for Depression: A New Approach to Preventing Relapse*, second edition, Guilford, New York, 2013.

Silverton, S. *The Mindfulness Breakthrough: The Revolutionary Approach to Dealing with Stress, Anxiety, and Depression*, Watkins, London, UK, 2012.

Singer, T. and Ricard, M. *Caring Economics: Conversations on Altruism and Compassion Between Scientists, Economists, and the Dalai Lama*, Picador, New York, 2015.

Smalley, S. L. and Winston, D. *Fully Present: The Science, Art, and Practice of Mindfulness*, DaCapo, Philadelphia, PA, 2010.

Stanley, S., Purser, R., and Singh, N. N. (eds). *Handbook of Ethical Foundations of Mindfulness*, Springer, New York, 2018.

Teasdale, J. D., Williams, M., and Segal, Z. V. *The Mindful Way Workbook: An Eight-Week Program to Free Yourself from Depression and Emotional Distress*, Guilford, New York, 2014.

Tolle, E. *The Power of Now*, New World Library, Novato, CA, 1999.

Treleaven, D. *Trauma-Sensitive Mindfulness: Practices for Safe and Transformative Healing*, W.W. Norton, New York, 2018.

Vo, D. X. *The Mindful Teen: Powerful Skills to Help You Handle Stress One Moment at a Time*, New Harbinger, Oakland, CA, 2015.

Wallace, B.A. *Tibetan Buddhism from the Ground Up*, Wisdom, Somerville, MA, 1993.

Williams, A. K., Owens, R., and Syedullah, J. *Radical Dharma: Talking Race, Love, and Liberation*, North Atlantic Books, Berkeley, 2016.

Williams, J.M.G., Teasdale, J. D., Segal, Z. V., and Kabat-Zinn, J. *The Mindful Way Through Depression: Freeing Yourself from Chronic Unhappiness*, Guilford, New York, 2007.

Williams, M. and Kabat-Zinn, J. (eds.). *Mindfulness: Diverse Perspectives on its Meaning, Origins, and Applications*, Routledge, Abingdon, UK, 2013.

Williams, M. and Penman, D. *Mindfulness: An Eight-Week Plan for Finding Peace in a Frantic World*, Rodale, New York, 2012.

Williams, M., Fennell, M., Barnhofeer, T., Crane, R., and Silverton, S. *Mindfulness and the Transformation of Despair: Working with People at Risk of Suicide*, Guilford, New York, 2015.

Wright, R. *Why Buddhism Is True: The Science and Philosophy of Meditation and Enlightenment*, Simon & Schuster, New York, 2017.

Yang, L. *Awakening Together: The Spiritual Practice of Inclusivity and Community*, Wisdom, Somerville, MA, 2017.

# Healing

Doidge, N. *The Brain's Way of Healing: Remarkable Discoveries and Recoveries from the Frontiers of Neuroplasticity*, Penguin Random House, New York, 2016.

Goleman, D. *Healing Emotions: Conversations with the Dalai Lama on Mindfulness, Emotions, and Health*, Shambhala, Boston, 1997.

Moyers, B. *Healing and the Mind*, Doubleday, New York, 1993.

Ornish, D. *Love and Survival: The Scientific Basis for the Healing Power of Intimacy*, HarperCollins, New York, 1998.

Remen, R. *Kitchen Table Wisdom: Stories that Heal*, Riverhead, New York, 1997.

Siegel, D. *The Mindful Brain: Reflection and Attunement in the Cultivation of Wellbeing*, W.W. Norton, New York, 2007.

Simmons, P. *Learning to Fall: The Blessings of an Imperfect Life*, Bantam, New York, 2002.

Tarrant, J. *The Light Inside the Dark: Zen, Soul, and the Spiritual Life*, HarperCollins, New York, 1998.

Tenzin Gyatso (the 14th Dalai Lama). *The Compassionate Life*, Wisdom, Boston, 2003.

Van der Kolk, B. *The Body Keeps the Score: Brain, Mind, and Body in the Healing of Trauma*, Penguin Random House, New York, 2014.

# Poetry

Eliot, T. S. *Four Quartets*, Harcourt Brace, New York, 1943, 1977.

Lao-Tzu, *Tao Te Ching*, (Stephen Mitchell, transl.), HarperCollins, New York, 1988.

Mitchell, S. *The Enlightened Heart*, Harper & Row, New York, 1989.

Oliver, M. *New and Selected Poems*, Beacon, Boston, 1992.

Tanahashi, K. and Leavitt, P. *The Complete Cold Mountain: Poems of the Legendary Hermit, Hanshan*, Shambhala, Boulder, CO, 2018.

Whyte, D. *The Heart Aroused: Poetry and the Preservation of the Soul in Corporate America*, Doubleday, New York, 1994.

# Other Books of Interest, Some Mentioned in the Text

Abram, D. *The Spell of the Sensuous*, Vintage, New York, 1996.

Ackerman, D. *A Natural History of the Senses*, Vintage, New York, 1990.

Blackburn, E. and Epel, E. *The Telomere Effect: A Revolutionary Approach to Living Younger, Healthier, Longer*, Grand Central Publishing, New York, 2017.

Bohm, D. *Wholeness and the Implicate Order*, Routledge and Kegan Paul, London, 1980.

Bryson, B. *A Short History of Nearly Everything*, Broadway, New York, 2003.

Carroll, S. *The Big Picture: On the Origins of Life, Meaning, and the Universe*, Dutton, New York, 2016.

Davidson, R. J., and Begley, S. *The Emotional Life of Your Brain*, Hudson St. Press, New York, 2012.

Glassman, B. *Bearing Witness: A Zen Master's Lessons in Making Peace*, Bell Tower, New York, 1998.

Greene, B. *The Elegant Universe*, Norton, New York, 1999.

Greene, B. *The Hidden Reality: Parallel Universes and the Deep Laws of the Cosmos*, Vintage, New York, 2011.

Harari, Y. N. *Homo Deus: A Brief History of Tomorrow*, HarperCollins, New York, 2017.

Harari, Y. N. *Sapiens: A Brief History of Humankind*, HarperCollins, New York, 2015.

Harari, Y. N. *21 Lessons for the 21st Century*, Penguin Random House, New York, 2018.

Hillman, J. *The Soul's Code: In Search of Character and Calling*, Random House, New York, 1996.

Holt, J. *When Einstein Walked with Gödel: Excursions to the Edge of Thought*, Farrar, Strauss & Giroux, New York, 2018.

Karr-Morse, R. and Wiley, M. S. *Ghosts from the Nursery: Tracing the Roots of Violence*, Atlantic Monthly Press, New York, 1997.

Katie, B. and Mitchell, S. *A Mind at Home with Itself*, HarperCollins, New York, 2017.

Kazanjian, V. H., and Laurence, P. L. (eds.). *Education as Transformation*, Peter Lang, New York, 2000.

Kurzweil, R. *The Age of Spiritual Machines*, Viking, New York, 1999.

Luke, H. *Old Age: Journey into Simplicity*, Parabola, New York, 1987.

Montague, A. *Touching: The Human Significance of the Skin*, Harper & Row, New York, 1978.

Nowak, M. and Highfield, M. A. *SuperCooperators: Altruism, Evolution, and Why We Need Each Other to Succeed*, Free Press, New York, 2011.

Palmer, P. *The Courage to Teach: Exploring the Inner Landscape of a Teacher's Life*, Jossey-Bass, San Francisco, 1998.

Pinker, S. *The Better Angels of Our Nature: Why Violence Has Declined*, Penguin Random House, New York, 2012.

Pinker, S. *Enlightenment Now: The Case for Reason, Science, Humanism, and Progress*, Penguin Random House, New York, 2018.

Pinker, S. *How the Mind Works*, W.W. Norton, New York, 1997.

Randall, L. *Knocking on Heaven's Door: How Physics and Scientific Thinking Illuminate the Universe and the Modern World*, HarperCollins, New York, 2011.

Randall, L. *Warped Passages: Unraveling the Mysteries of the Universe's Hidden Dimensions*, Ecco, HarperCollins, New York, 2005.

Ravel, J.-F. and Ricard, M. *The Monk and the Philosopher: A Father and Son Discuss the Meaning of Life*, Schocken, New York, 1998.

Ricard, M. *Altruism: The Power of Compassion to Change Yourself and the World*, Little Brown, New York, 2013.

Ryan, T. *A Mindful Nation: How a Simple Practice Can Help Us Reduce Stress, Improve Performance, and Recapture the American Spirit*, Hay House, New York, 2012.

Sachs, J. D. *The Price of Civilization: Reawakening American Virtue and Prosperity*, Random House, New York, 2011.

Sachs, O. *The Man Who Mistook His Wife for a Hat*, Touchstone, New York, 1970.

Sachs, O. *The River of Consciousness*, Knopf, New York, 2017.

Sapolsky, R. *Behave: The Biology of Humans at Our Best and Worst*, Penguin Random House, New York, 2017.

Schwartz, J. M. and Begley, S. *The Mind and the Brain: Neuroplasticity and the Power of Mental Force*, HarperCollins, New York, 2002.

Singh, S. *Fermat's Enigma*, Anchor, New York, 1997.

Tanahashi, K. *The Heart Sutra: A Comprehensive Guide to the Classic of Mahayana Buddhism*, Shambhala, Boulder, CO, 2016.

Tegmark, M. *Life 3.0: Being Human in the Age of Artificial Intelligence*, Knopf, New York, 2017.

Tegmark, M. *The Mathematical Universe: My Quest for the Ultimate Nature of Reality*, Random House, New York, 2014.

Turkle, S. *Alone Together: Why We Expect More from Technology and Less from Each Other*, Basic Books, New York, 2011.

Turkle, S. *Reclaiming Conversation: The Power of Talk in a Digital Age*, Penguin Random House, New York, 2015.

Varela, F. J., Thompson, E., and Rosch, E. *The Embodied Mind: Cognitive Science and Human Experience*, revised edition, MIT Press, Cambridge, MA, 2016.

# Websites

| | |
|---|---|
| www.umassmed.edu/cfm | Website of the Center for Mindfulness, UMass Medical School |
| www.brown.edu/academics/public -health/research/mindfulness/home | Website of the Mindfulness Center at Brown University |
| www.mindandlife.org | Website of the Mind and Life Institute |
| www.dharma.org | Vipassana retreat centers and schedules |

CREDITS AND PERMISSIONS
(for all four books in the series)

Basho, three-line poem "Old pond," translated by Michael Katz, from *The Enlightened Heart: An Anthology of Sacred Poetry,* edited by Stephen Mitchell (New York: Harper & Row, 1989). Reprinted with the permission of the translator. "Even in Kyoto" from *The Essential Haiku: Versions of Basho, Buson, and Issa,* translated and edited by Robert Hass. Copyright © 1994 by Robert Hass. Reprinted with the permission of HarperCollins Publishers, Inc.

Sandra Blakeslee, excerpts from "Exercising Toward Repair of the Spinal Cord" from *The Sunday New York Times* (September 22, 2002). Copyright © 2002 by The New York Times Company. Reprinted with permission.

Buddha, excerpt from *The Middle Length Discourses of the Buddha,* translated by Bikkhu Nanamoi and Bikkhu Bodhi. Copyright © 1995 by Bikkhu Nanamoi and Bikkhu Bodhi. Reprinted with the permission of Wisdom Publications, 199 Elm Street, Somerville, MA 02144, USA, www.wisdompubs.org.

Chuang Tzu, excerpt from "The Empty Boat," translated by Thomas Merton, from *The Collected Poems of Thomas Merton.* Copyright © 1965 by The Abbey of Gethsemani. Reprinted with the permission of New Directions Publishing Corporation.

Definition for "sentient" from *American Heritage Dictionary of the English Language, Third Edition.* Copyright © 2000 by Houghton Mifflin Company. Reprinted with the permission of Houghton Mifflin Company.

Emily Dickinson, "I'm Nobody! Who are you?", "Me from Myself to banish," and excerpt from "I dwell in possibility" from *The Complete Poems of Emily*

*Dickinson,* edited by Thomas H. Johnson. Copyright © 1945, 1951, 1955, 1979, 1983 by the President and Fellows of Harvard College. Reprinted with the permission of The Belknap Press of Harvard University Press.

T. S. Eliot, excerpts from "Burnt Norton," "Little Gidding," and "East Coker" from *Four Quartets.* Copyright © 1936 by Harcourt, Inc., renewed © 1964 by T. S. Eliot. Reprinted with the permission of Harcourt, Inc. and Faber and Faber Ltd.

Thomas Friedman, excerpts from "Foreign Affairs; Cyber-Serfdom" from *The New York Times* (January 30, 2001). Copyright © 2001 by The New York Times Company. Reprinted with permission.

Goethe, excerpt from *The Rag and Bone Shop of the Heart: Poems for Men,* edited by Robert Bly et al. Copyright © 1992 by Robert Bly. Reprinted with the permission of HarperCollins Publishers, Inc. Excerpt from "The Holy Longing" from *News of the Universe* (Sierra Club Books, 1980). Copyright © 1980 by Robert Bly. Reprinted with the permission of the translator.

Excerpts from "Heart Sutra" from *Chanting with English Translations* (Cumberland, RI: Kwan Um Zen School, 1983). Reprinted with the permission of The Kwan Um School of Zen.

Juan Ramon Jiménez, "Oceans" and "I am not I" from *Selected Poems of Lorca and Jiménez,* chosen and translated by Robert Bly (Boston: Beacon Press, 1973). Copyright © 1973 by Robert Bly. Reprinted with the permission of the translator.

Kabir, excerpts from *The Kabir Book: Forty-four of the Ecstatic Poems of Kabir,* versions by Robert Bly (Boston: Beacon Press, 1977). Copyright © 1977 by Robert Bly. Reprinted with the permission of Robert Bly.

Lao Tzu, excerpts from *Tao Te Ching,* translated by Stephen Mitchell. Copyright © 1988 by Stephen Mitchell. Reprinted with the permission of HarperCollins Publishers, Inc.

Antonio Machado, excerpt from "The wind one brilliant day," translated by Robert Bly, from *Times Alone: Selected Poems of Antonio Machado* (Middletown, CT: Wesleyan University Press, 1983). Copyright © 1983 by Robert Bly. Reprinted with the permission of the translator.

Naomi Shihab Nye, "Kindness" from *Words Under the Words: Selected Poems* (Portland, OR: Eighth Mountain Press, 1995). Copyright © 1995 by Naomi Shihab Nye. Reprinted with the permission of the author.

Mary Oliver, "The Summer Day" from *New and Selected Poems*. Copyright © 1992 by Mary Oliver. Reprinted with the permission of Beacon Press, Boston. "Lingering in Happiness" from *Why I Wake Early*. Copyright © 2004 by Mary Oliver. Reprinted with the permission of Beacon Press, Boston. "The Journey" from *Dream Work*. Copyright © 1986 by Mary Oliver. Reprinted with the permission of Grove/Atlantic, Inc.

Matt Richtel, excerpts from "The Lure of Data: Is it Addictive?" from *The New York Times* (July 6, 2003). Copyright © 2003 by The New York Times Company. Reprinted by permission.

Rainer Maria Rilke, "My life is not this steeply sloping hour" from *Selected Poems of Rainer Maria Rilke* (New York: Harper, 1981). Copyright © 1981 by Robert Bly. Reprinted with the permission of the translator.

Jelaluddin Rumi, excerpt ["Outside, the freezing desert night. / This other night grows warm, kindling..."], translated by Coleman Barks with John Moyne, from *The Enlightened Heart: An Anthology of Sacred Poetry*, edited by Stephen Mitchell (New York: Harper & Row, 1989). Copyright © by Coleman Barks. "The Guest House" and excerpt from "No Room for Form" from *The Essential Rumi*, translated by Coleman Barks with John Moyne. Copyright © 1995 by Coleman Barks. Excerpt ["Today like every other day / We wake up empty and scared..."] translated by Coleman Barks (previously unpublished). All reprinted with the permission of Coleman Barks.

Ryokan, poem translated by John Stevens from *One Robe, One Bowl*. Copyright © 1977 by John Stevens. Reprinted with the permission of Shambhala Publications, Inc.

Antoine de Saint-Exupéry, excerpt from *The Little Prince*. Copyright © 1943 by Antoine de Saint-Exupéry. Reprinted with the permission of Harcourt, Inc.

Seng-Ts'an, excerpts from *Hsin-hsin Ming: Verses on the Faith-Mind*, translated by Richard B. Clarke. Copyright © 1973, 1984, 2001 by Richard B. Clarke. Reprinted with the permission of White Pine Press, Buffalo, NY, www.whitepine.org.

William Stafford, "You Reading This, Be Ready" from *The Way It Is: New and Selected Poems*. Copyright © 1998 by the Estate of William Stafford. Reprinted with the permission of Graywolf Press, St. Paul, MN. "Being a Person." Copyright © by William Stafford. Reprinted with the permission of Kim Stafford.

Tenzin Gyatso, excerpt from *The Compassionate Life*. Copyright © 2001 by Tenzin Gyatso. Reprinted with the permission of Wisdom Publications, 199 Elm Street, Somerville, MA 02144, USA, www.wisdompubs.org.

Tung-Shan, excerpt ["If you look for the truth outside yourself, / It gets farther and farther away..."], translated by Stephen Mitchell, from *The Enlightened Heart: An Anthology of Sacred Poetry*, edited by Stephen Mitchell. Copyright © 1989 by Stephen Mitchell. Reprinted with the permission of HarperCollins Publishers, Inc.

Derek Walcott, "Love After Love" from *Collected Poems 1948–1984*. Copyright © 1986 by Derek Walcott. Reprinted with the permission of Farrar, Straus & Giroux, LLC.

David Whyte, "Sweet Darkness" from *Fire in the Earth*. Copyright © 1992 by David Whyte. Reprinted with the permission of Many Rivers Press, Langley, WA. "Enough" from *Where Many Rivers Meet*. Copyright © 2000 by David Whyte. Reprinted with the permission of Many Rivers Press, Langley, WA. Excerpt from *Crossing the Unknown Sea: Work as a Pilgrimage of Identity.* Copyright © 2001 by David Whyte. Reprinted with the permission of Riverhead Books, a division of Penguin Group (USA) Inc.

William Carlos Williams, excerpt from "Asphodel, That Greeny Flower" (Book I) ["My heart rouses / thinking to bring you news / of something / that concerns you..."] from *The Collected Poems of William Carlos Williams, Volume II, 1939–1962,* edited by Christopher MacGowan. Copyright © 1944 by William Carlos Williams. Reprinted with the permission of New Directions Publishing Corporation.

William Butler Yeats, excerpts from "Gratitude to the Unknown Instructors," "Sailing to Byzantium," and "Broken Dreams" from *The Poems of W. B. Yeats: A New Edition,* edited by Richard J. Finneran. Copyright © 1933 by Macmillan Publishing Company, renewed © 1961 by Georgie Yeats. Reprinted with the permission of Simon & Schuster Adult Publishing.

# INDEX

*Page references in italics indicate quotes or poetry citations.*

# ABOUT THE AUTHOR

JON KABAT-ZINN, Ph.D., is the founder of MBSR (mindfulness-based stress reduction) and the Stress Reduction Clinic (1979) and of the Center for Mindfulness in Medicine, Health Care, and Society (1995) at the University of Massachusetts Medical School. He is also professor of Medicine emeritus. He leads workshops and retreats on mindfulness for health professionals, the tech and business communities, and for lay audiences worldwide. He is a strong proponent of social justice and economic justice. He is the author or coauthor of fourteen books, including the bestselling *Wherever You Go, There You Are* and *Full Catastrophe Living*. With his wife Myla Kabat-Zinn, he published a book on mindful parenting, *Everyday Blessings*. He has been featured in numerous documentaries for television around the world, including the PBS Special *Healing and the Mind* with Bill Moyers, *Oprah*, and CBS's *60 Minutes* with Anderson Cooper. He lives in Massachusetts. His work has contributed to a growing movement of mindfulness into mainstream institutions such as medicine, psychology, health care, neuroscience, schools, higher education, business, social justice, criminal justice, prisons, the law, technology, government, and professional sports. Hospitals and medical centers around the world now offer clinical programs based on training in mindfulness and MBSR.

Continue the journey and get the full set of
Jon Kabat-Zinn's four small-but-mighty guides to
mindfulness and meditation, as well as his
bestselling classic *Wherever You Go, There You Are.*

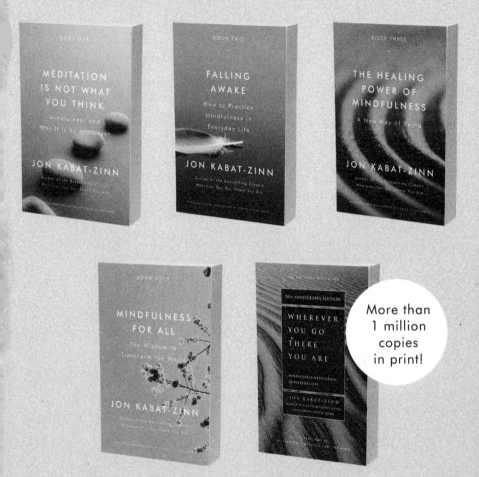

**JON KABAT-ZINN, PhD,** is the founder of Mindfulness-Based
Stress Reduction (MBSR) and of the Center for Mindfulness in Medicine,
Health Care and Society at the University of Massachusetts, where he
is Professor of Medicine emeritus. He is the author of numerous bestselling books about mindfulness and meditation. For more information,
visit www.jonkabat-zinn.com.

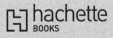
hachette
BOOKS

*Guided Mindfulness Meditation Practices with Jon Kabat-Zinn*

**Obtainable as apps, downloads, or CDs**
**(see below for links)**

## Series 1

These guided meditations (the body scan and sitting meditation) and guided mindful yoga practices 1 and 2 form the foundational practices of MBSR and are used in MBSR programs around the world. These practices and their use are described in detail in *Full Catastrophe Living*. Each meditation is 45 minutes in length.

## Series 2

These guided meditations are designed for people who want a range of shorter guided meditations to help them develop and/or expand and deepen a personal meditation practice based on mindfulness. The series includes the mountain and lake meditations (each 20 minutes) as well as a range of other 10-minute, 20-minute, and 30-minute sitting and lying down practices. This series was originally developed to accompany *Wherever You Go, There You Are*.

## Series 3

These guided meditations are designed to accompany this book and the other three volumes based on *Coming to Our Senses*. Series 3 includes guided meditations on the breath and body sensations (breathscape and bodyscape), on sounds (soundscape), thoughts and emotions (mindscape), choiceless awareness (nowscape), and lovingkindness (heartscape), as well as instructions for lying down meditation (corpse pose/dying before you die), mindful walking, and cultivating mindfulness in everyday life (lifescape).

**For iPhone and Android apps:** www.mindfulnessapps.com

**For digital downloads:** www.betterlisten.com/pages/jonkabatzinnseries123

**For CD sets:** www.soundstrue.com/jon-kabat-zinn